Spinal Cord Injury Medicine

Spinal Cord Injury Medicine

Edited by Garrett Donovan

hayle medical

New York

Hayle Medical,
750 Third Avenue, 9ᵗʰ Floor,
New York, NY 10017, USA

Visit us on the World Wide Web at:
www.haylemedical.com

ISBN: 978-1-63241-673-5

Cataloging-in-Publication Data

Spinal cord injury medicine / edited by Garrett Donovan.
p. cm.
Includes bibliographical references and index.
ISBN 978-1-63241-673-5
1. Spinal cord--Wounds and injuries. 2. Spinal cord--Wounds and injuries--Diagnosis.
3. Spinal cord--Wounds and injuries--Treatment. I. Donovan, Garrett.
RD594.3 .S74 2019
617.482 075 7--dc23

Table of Contents

Preface

Over the recent decade, advancements and applications have progressed exponentially. This has led to the increased interest in this field and projects are being conducted to enhance knowledge. The main objective of this book is to present some of the critical challenges and provide insights into possible solutions. This book will answer the varied questions that arise in the field and also provide an increased scope for furthering studies.

A spinal cord injury (SCI) is the damage to the spinal cord, which leads to permanent or temporary changes in its function. Most cases of SCI occur due to physical traumas including gunshots, sports injuries, car accidents, tumors, infection, etc. It is characterized by a loss of muscle function, autonomic function or sensation in different parts of the body, particularly in the areas below the level of the injury. Depending on the injury, damage can extend into a state between paralysis and incontinence. SCI patients need to undergo extended periods of care. However, even with the best possible treatment, SCI generally results in some incurable impairment. There has been tremendous research in the treatment of these injuries such as stem cell implantation, epidural spinal stimulation, engineered materials for tissue support and wearable robotic exoskeletons. This book is a compilation of chapters that discuss the most vital concepts and emerging trends in the field of spinal cord injury medicine. It aims to shed light on some of the unexplored aspects of spinal cord injuries and the recent researches in their medical management. For all those who are interested in this field, this book can prove to be an essential guide.

I hope that this book, with its visionary approach, will be a valuable addition and will promote interest among readers. Each of the authors has provided their extraordinary competence in their specific fields by providing different perspectives as they come from diverse nations and regions. I thank them for their contributions.

Editor

Role of Gait Training in Recovery of Standing and Walking in Subjects with Spinal Cord Injury

Mokhtar Arazpour, Guive Sharifi,
Mohammad Ebrahim Mousavi and Maryam Maleki

Abstract

Gait training has an important role in rehabilitation of standing and walking in spinal cord injury (SCI) patients. There were different types of gait training in these subjects. Both the body weight support treadmill training and robotic-assisted and robotic exoskeleton are effective and secure methods for gait training and improving the energy demand and metabolic cost in SCI patients in different level of injury. The powered exoskeletons can provide patients with SCI the ability to walk with the lowest energy consumption. The powered exoskeleton's energy consumption and speed of walking depend on the training duration. Based on different types of gait training methods, training time, and other affected parameters, the aim of this chapter was to evaluate the role of gait training in recovery of standing and walking in SCI patients.

Keywords: spinal cord injury, gait training, standing, walking

1. Introduction

The act of learning how to walk (as a child, or more frequently, after sustaining an injury or disability) is so-called **gait training** or **gait rehabilitation**. In this chapter, we focus on gait training after spinal cord injury (SCI). The purpose of gait training for subjects with SCI is usually to increase walking endurance and to decrease subject's dependency. Standing and walking can help to prevent contractures of the lower limb joints, as well as osteoporosis, spasticity, bed sores and edema, complete discharge of bladder, and prevention of bladder infection in subjects with SCI [1–4].

Spinal cord injury is spinal cord damaging that causes changes in function, most frequently and importantly, disruption in lower limb motor and sensation. Inability to walk is the most important limitation for affected patients [5]. Among lots of serious problem which patients encounter with, but after injury the first question is "will I ever walk again?" [6]. As a result, retraining the affected patients to achieve walking ability is important.

The main determinants of normal gait are [7]:

- Stability and posture,

- Range of motion (ROM),

- Muscle strength,

- Co-ordinated motor control,

- Muscle tone,

- Proprioception,

- Vision,

- Cognition,

- Aerobic capacity out of which the first six factors are impaired in spinal cord injured individuals.

In patients with SCI, there are no main determinants of normal gait, but in recent years, there have been advancements in how the patients can increase the ability to walk. Rehabilitation procedures should focus on the development of outcome by using the neuroplasticity and by using a functional training.

Lovely et al. in 1990 demonstrated neuronal circuits below the level of lesion become activated by an appropriate afferent input. They established that stepping practice plays an important role in training [8]. When the practice of stepping is accomplished, walking can be done more effective than when it is not practiced. In spinal cord, when a motor task wants to be recognized in neural circuit, it should be practiced appropriately and sufficiently. The name of this process is training [9]. De Leon et al. in 1998 and Wirz et al., 2001 stated that appropriate afferent input activate neuronal networks below the level of injury in a SCI patients, and activated neural network generate electromyography activity for suitable function (even in complete SCI without supraspinal input) [10, 11]. Dietz et al. in different experiments in human and animals revealed externally assisted walking, with tools and equipment or therapist, when appropriate afferent input will drive to spinal cord, a locomotor pattern will train and muscle activity (EMG) will be turned on even in complete SCI; however, muscle activity in complete SCI is low in comparison with healthy subjects but muscle EMG will increase by practicing more and more during training sessions [12].

One of the important afferent inputs is foot load receptor input. Researchers perceive the importance of these kinds of afferent input when they use externally assisted walking while patients are unloading. In this experiment, they understand unloading does not activate muscle EMG activity and they claim that, body unloading and reloading are considered to be of crucial importance to convince training effects upon the neurological locomotor centers,

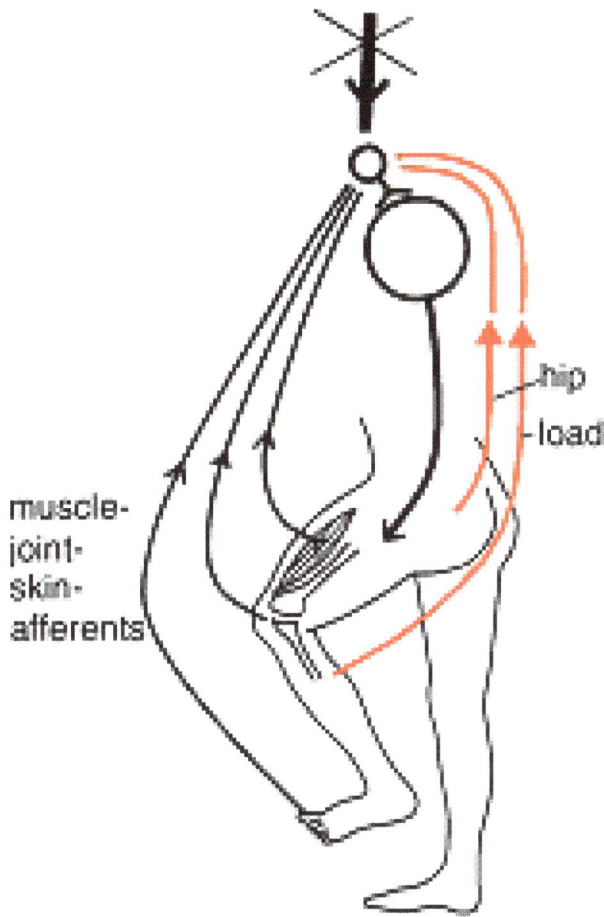

Figure 1. Schematic drawing of the afferent input from load- and hip joint [14].

because the afferent input from foot pressure during the stance phase is essential for the activation of spinal neuronal network (**Figure 1**) [13]. Dietz in 2008 suggested that another important input after foot contact pressure is proprioceptive input from extensor hip muscles. Foot sole mechanoreceptor with hip extensor muscles proprioception provides load information (**Figure 1**) [13].

2. Gait rehabilitation interventions following spinal cord injury

Until now, many therapeutic strategies have been developed for promoting locomotor activity of SCI subjects ranged from those that compensate for weakened or lost function (e.g. orthotic gait training) to strategies based on the concepts of central nervous system (CNS) plasticity (e.g. Erigo therapy and body weight–supported tread mill training) [15, 16]. Strategies that are based on the concept of CNS plasticity have shown improvement and enhancement in walking ability of SCI subjects through implementing the task-specific sensory input and repetitive and intensive gait therapy [17, 18]. These strategies will be explained as following.

3. Early gait rehabilitation interventions after spinal cord injury (Erigo therapy)

SCI subjects, in acute stages, are disposed to orthostatic hypotension occurrences while transferred from a horizontal to an upright position due to the lack of sympathetic activity and also leg muscle contractions that finally lead to delay in starting the functional gait training [18, 19]. On the other hand, the mobilization and verticalization of SCI patients in acute care with limited or no capacity for cooperation can be very challenging. One approach to decrease the orthostatic hypotension incidences is utilizing tilt table. Many limitations related to the use of traditional tilt table have been reported such as no leg movements, limited training duration due to the lack of patient's cardiovascular stability and excessive labor load on therapist for passive movements. Therefore, for overcoming of such limitations a novel, robotic tilt table so-called Erigo was designed and developed, which offered a locomotion therapy at a very early stage of rehabilitation. These types of approaches through utilizing a safe mobilization and intensive sensorimotor stimulation, ambulates the lower extremity, and suggests a wide range of positive impacts and functions to enhance early rehabilitation of SCI patients [18–20].

The design and construction of the "Erigo" was based on the conventional tilt table but combines gradual verticalization plus robotic leg movement's therapy and functional electrical stimulation [18] (**Figure 2**). The main superiority of "Erigo" to the traditional tilt table was utilizing the robotic leg movement and the cyclic leg loading that produce critical afferent stimuli for the central nervous system [18, 20, 21]. These afferent stimuli result in muscle activation, improved muscle pump function and venous return, which eventually result in improved cardiovascular stability in SCI subjects. There are a few studies about the efficacy of "Erigo" following spinal cord injury [18, 22, 23]. According to the previous research by Colombo et al., using Novel tilt table (tilted to 60° upright position) in five subjects with complete SCI (ASIA impairment scale A between C4 and C7) resulted in the increase of blood pressure and after stopping the automated movement, the mean arterial pressure decreased statistically significant($P < 0.0001$) [14]. Although this study showed the positive effects of passive movements of leg through using "Erigo" therapy on circulatory system in SCI patients, it has to be stated that further studies are necessary to test this type of approach in a larder patients group of SCI with different level of injury and also in the long term to indicate the direct effects of "Erigo" therapy.

Also Laubacher et al. indicated that the "Erigo" therapy is practical for respiratory and cardiopulmonary training and evaluation of incomplete SCI subjects and they found it was a tolerable and implementable approach [22]. Another approach in the rehabilitation of SCI subjects is combining the tilt table with vibrating foot plates (whole-body vibration) that focus on the activation of muscular and vascular systems. Herrero et al., found that whole body vibration (WBV) is an effective approach to enhance leg blood flow and to stimulate muscle activity in SCI subjects; therefore, they concluded that this approach could be incorporated in the rehabilitation programs of SCI subjects. So in future studies, we need to compare the efficacy of Erigo therapy and whole body vibration (WBV) on orthostatic, blood pressure, and EMG in subjects with SCI [24].

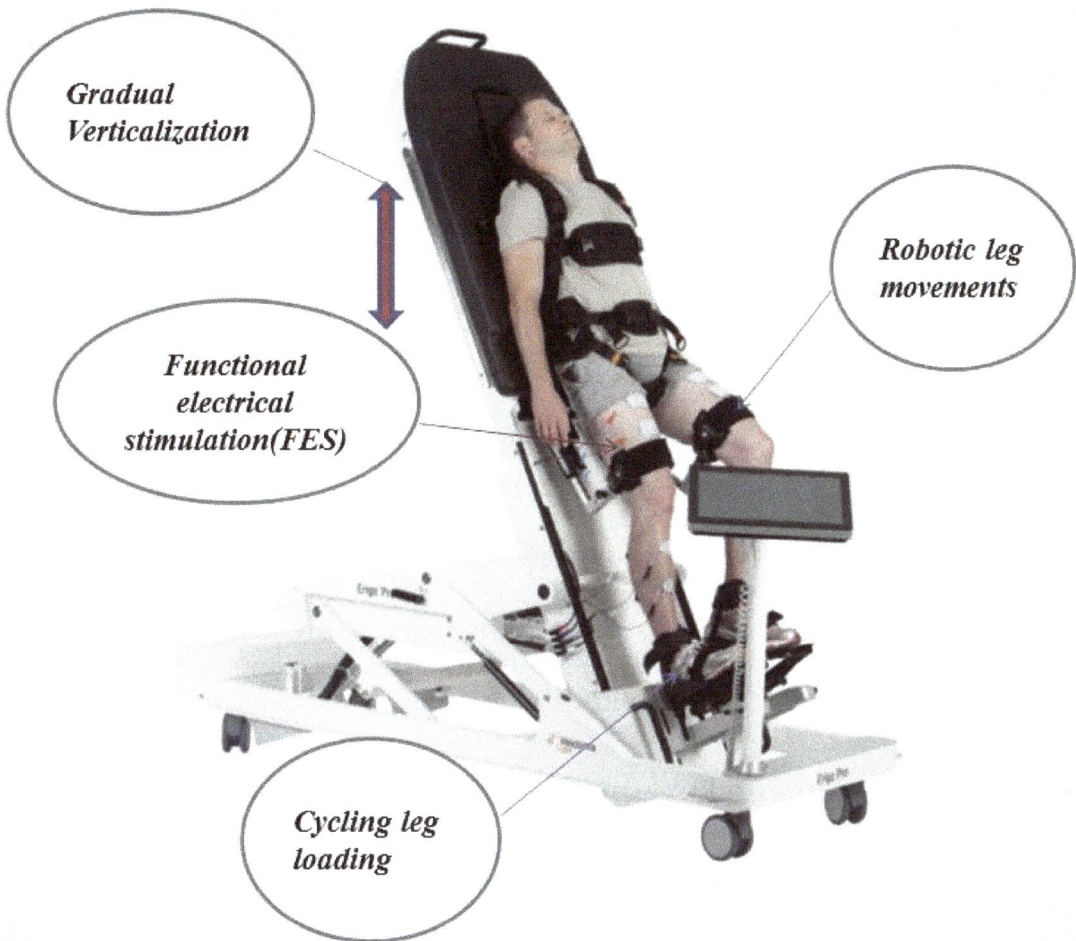

Figure 2. Erigo components.

Also integrating functional electrical stimulation (FES) into "Erigo" provides more physiological and clinical benefits (**Figure 3**). The nerve endings are stimulated through attaching electrodes to the skin, which results in contraction and activation of muscles. Many positive effects have been reported by using of "Erigo" plus FES like improving in the cardiovascular system and metabolism condition, decreasing spasticity, improving the muscle tone, reducing long-term consequences due to the lack of muscle activity, inducing functional movements, increasing cardiovascular stability during upright position, and promoting the orthostatic tolerance by enhancing venous return in individual with SCI [18, 22, 25, 26]. Thrasher et al. compared the effects of isometric FES and dynamic FES on cardiovascular parameters on an active tilt-table stepper in 16 young and healthy adults. They stated that isometric FES led to short-term increases in blood pressure and also heart rate, but dynamic FES maintained increase in blood pressure over the long term. They postulated that however FES has potential to counteract orthostatic stress it should be combined with movements of leg [27]. In a pilot study, Yoshida et al. found that through applying FES cyclically to the leg muscles of 10 SCI subjects at T6 or higher, they could better retain their blood pressure. Although FES and

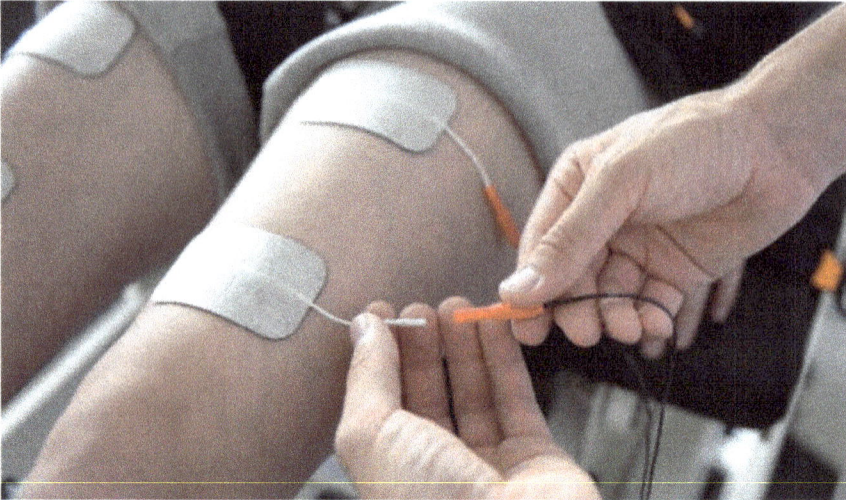

Figure 3. Functional electrical stimulation synchronized with leg cycling in "Erigo".

passive stepping by Erigo achieves this function by inducing venous return, passive stepping was less effective than FES in this study [23]. Finally, many studies are needed to extend these findings to the community of people with SCI with different levels of injury.

4. Body weight–supported treadmill training approaches after spinal cord injury

The most outstanding strategy for regaining the walking ability in SCI subjects is body weight–supported treadmill training (BWSTT) [16, 26, 28]. Traditionally, BWSTT device supported some of the SCI patient's body weight by using a harness, as therapists manually assist their legs via the stepping movement on a treadmill. Although, it has been shown that such interventions could enhance and promote locomotor activity in SCI subjects, according to the previous researches, traditional gait therapy had many disadvantages such as excessive labor load on therapists, confined training duration, and gait pattern without any feedback for patients (**Figure 4**) [17]. Therefore, body weight–supported treadmill training using lower extremity robotic exoskeleton (e.g. Lokomat) was designed and developed and initially implemented for SCI rehabilitation. The BWSTT with robotics exoskeleton has originated from the central pattern generator (CPG) and is a secure and functional intervention that allows gait training by covering the limitations of conventional gait therapy [16, 29].

One of the famous robotics exoskeleton use in conjunction with the BWSTT is the Lokomat (Hocoma AG, Volketswil, Switzerland), which is a bilateral robotic orthosis, worn by patients, and attaches to a treadmill frame to provide powered assistance at the hip and knee in the sagittal plane, while a therapist can check the system and regulate assistance as necessary (**Figure 5**) [17, 28].

The Lokomat has been demonstrated to be effective in producing more normal walking patterns and promoting walking ability in subjects with incomplete SCI. Generally, applying the robotic

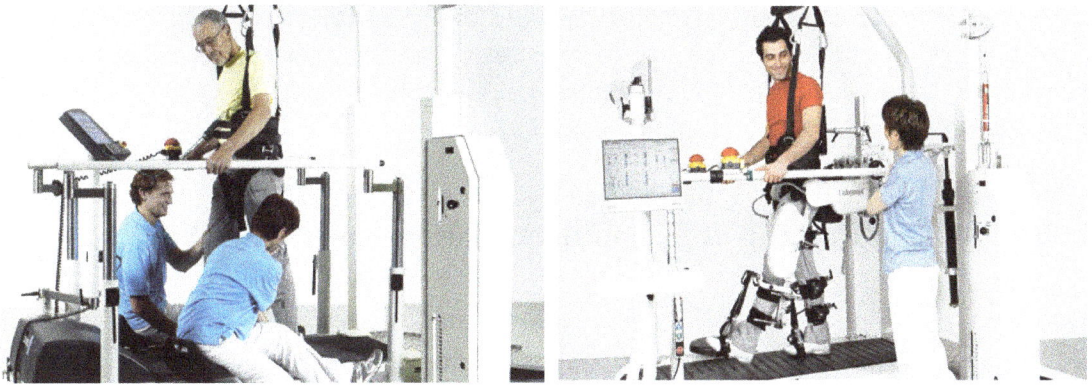

Figure 4. Traditional BWSTT (A) V.S. BWSTT plus robotic exoskeleton (B).

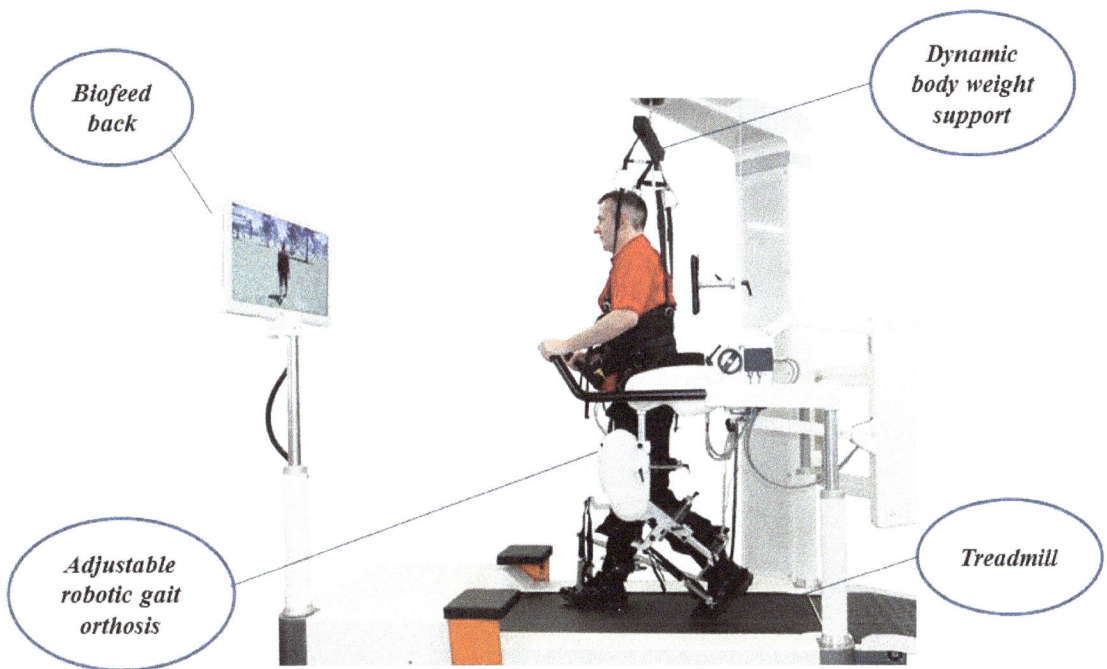

Figure 5. Lokomat components.

exoskeleton device in conjunction with the BWSTT, in gait rehabilitation procedure, could potentially accelerate recovery of walking ability in individual following SCI through enhancing the duration of training and reducing the labor load on physical therapists [17, 28, 29].

5. Orthotic gait training

There are different types of orthoses and assistive devices for standing and walking in complete and incomplete spinal cord injury subjects [30]. This type of intervention ranged from solid ankle foot orthosis to reciprocating gait orthoses and powered gait orthoses, which were used to low incomplete level of spinal cord injury and high complete or incomplete level of injury [31]. In general concept, all orthoses were used with walking aid for ambulation. Several factors influenced the providing walking ability via orthoses in the SCI subjects, which gait training is the important of them [32].

6. Orthotic gait training of SCI subjects with the mechanical orthoses

There were different types of mechanical orthoses such as hip-knee-ankle-foot orthosis, reciprocating gait orthosis (RGO) (**Figure 6**), hip guidance orthosis, and medial linkage orthoses (e.g. walkabout orthosis (WO), Primewalk orthosis (**Figure 7**)) to provide standing and walking in subjects with SCI [30]. Several studies evaluated this type of orthoses on walking ability in these subjects [30]. Based on the evaluation of the energy expenditure, Harvey et al. demonstrated that energy consumption of walking with the WO were greater than walking with the isocentric reciprocating gait orthosis (IRGO) in SCI subjects with T9–12 paraplegia [33]. In addition in another study, Harvey et al. demonstrated that stand up and sit down with WO was easier than IRGO, but IRGO provided faster and more independent ambulation [34]. In comparison of the attitude of subjects with SCI when using WO and the IRGO, Harvey et al. reported few

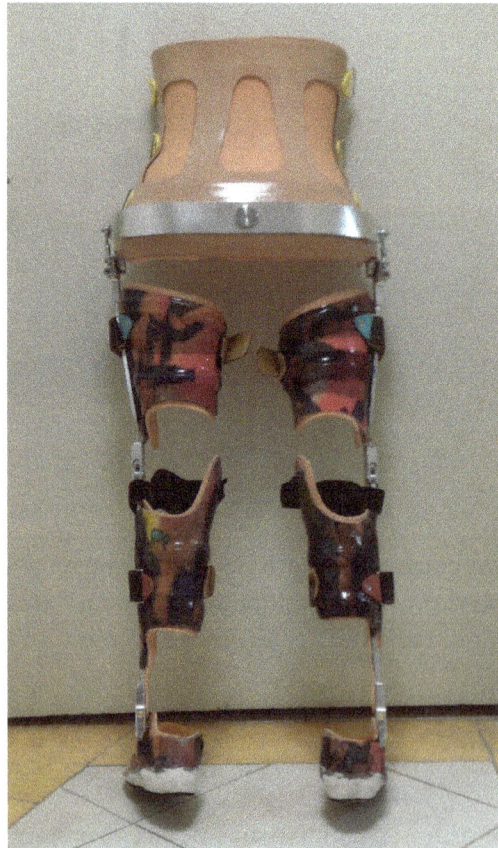

Figure 6. Isocentric reciprocating gait orthosis [32].

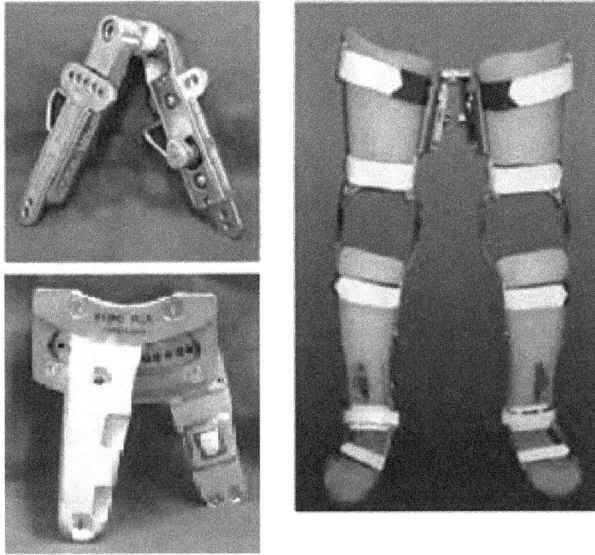

Figure 7. Walkabout orthosis and Primewalk orthosis.

subjects used orthosis more than once every 2 weeks, and SCI individuals were primarily wearing the orthoses for therapeutic aims [35]. To evaluate the influence of Primewalk orthosis and walkabout orthosis in improving the walking performance in subjects with SCI, Ongio et al. demonstrated the Primewalk orthosis had better effect in walking efficiency than that of the Walkabout orthosis [36].

Training time announced different in this field between 2 until 12 weeks. Longitudinal training program demonstrated the better results on the improvement of walking parameters. The maximum rate of the speed of walking reported from 0.13 to 0.63 m/s, which is 13–57% of the optimal speed (1.1 m/s) required for successful community ambulation [37]. Home or indoor mobility for exercise, upright posture, and standing reported final benefits of orthotics gait rehabilitation [38, 39].

The successful orthotic gait rehabilitation in SCI subjects related to the several factors included well-motivated, with complete level of injury at T9 or below, incomplete level of injury, postural control, and [39–41] good upper extremity strength, as well as less spasticity and low level contractures [42], reduced thoracolumbar mobility, back pain, or any musculoskeletal problems that influenced standing upright [33, 43]. Orthotic gait rehabilitation can be influenced by the acceptance of orthoses. In other words, acceptance of orthoses may be influenced by donning and doffing time, the best time for donning and doffing of orthosis should be less than 5 minutes [31].

7. Orthotic gait training of SCI subjects with powered gait orthoses

Providing gait training in different environments such as clinic, home, or community announced as the main benefit of wearing powered gait orthosis [3]. Only limited PGOs are currently commercially available to the public and therefore would be able to be used

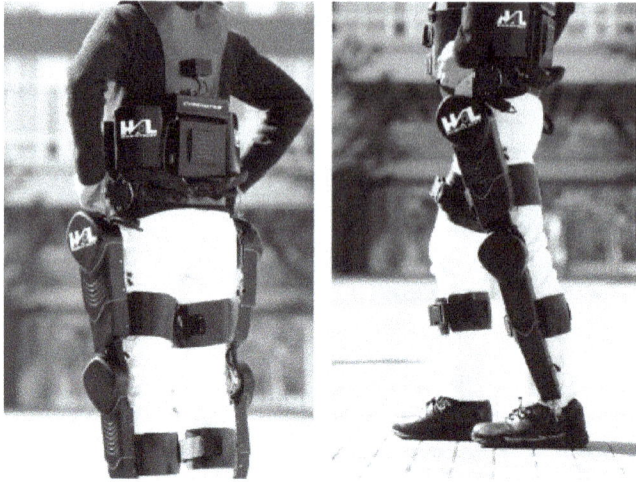

Figure 8. The HAL-5 type-C (hybrid assistive limb).

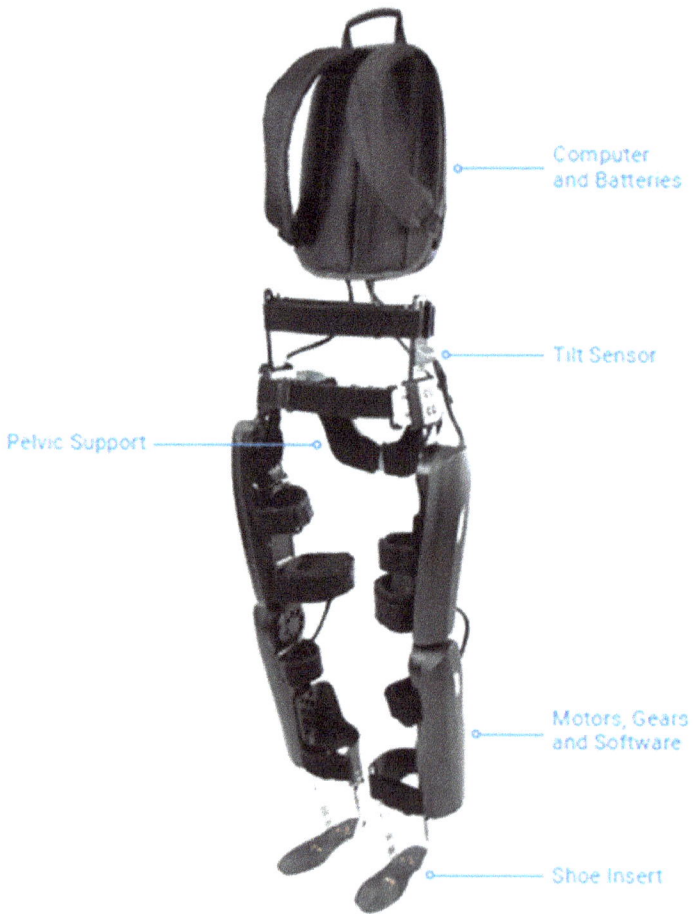

Computer and Batteries

Tilt Sensor

Pelvic Support

Motors, Gears and Software

Shoe Insert

Figure 9. The ReWalk powered orthosis (Argo Medical Technologies).

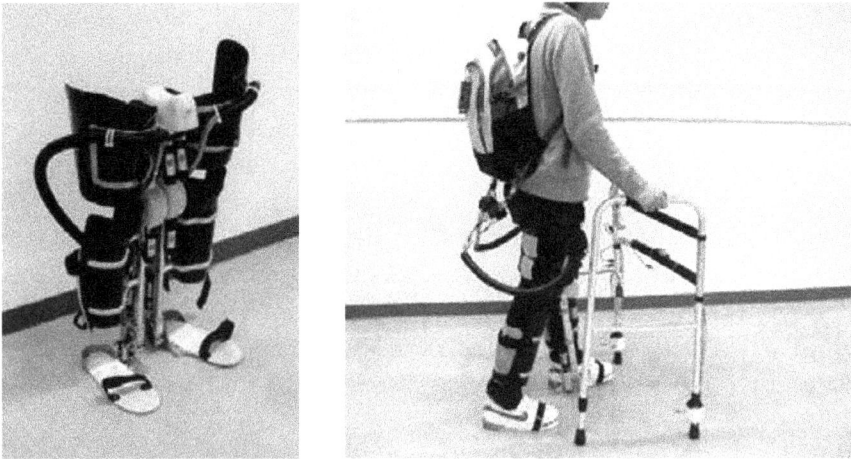

Figure 10. The wearable power assist locomotor.

in the field in SCI subjects. The concept of using PGOs is the reduction of energy demand in uses and reduces loads on the upper limb joints.

The HAL-5 Type-C (hybrid assistive limb) (**Figure 8**), the ReWalk powered orthosis (Argo Medical Technologies) (**Figure 9**), the wearable power assist locomotor (**Figure 10**), and the eLEGS-powered orthosis (Berkeley Bionics) (**Figure 11**) are commercially powered orthoses for ambulation in SCI subjects.

In the evaluation of the gait training with the HAL-6LB on the SCI subject for 8 days, for 2 hours per day, Tsukahara et al. reported that walking speed and cadence were 0.11 m/s and

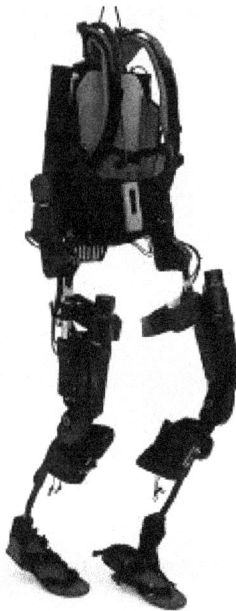

Figure 11. The eLEGS-powered orthosis (Berkeley Bionics).

20 steps/minutes, respectively [44]. In the evaluation of Rewalk exoskeleton on safety and tolerance in SCI patients, Zeilig et al. reported that mean time to walk 10 m was 47 seconds following training when using the Rewalk [45]. In another study, distance walked for 50–100 m announced between 5 and 10 minutes continually. The mean walking speed was 0.25 m/s [46]. In the evaluation of the wearable power assist locomotor orthosis (WPAL) on walking, physiological cost index (PCI) and muscle activity of the upper extremities in SCI subjects, Tanabe et al. reported all patients walked independently with the new powered device. The increased walking duration and distance of walking and reduction of the PCI and muscle activity of upper limbs with the WPAL compared to that the Primewalk orthosis [47]. Based on the literature in this field, we can conclude that PGOs can enable safe walking and reduce energy expenditure compared to mechanical orthoses in SCI subjects.

8. Orthotic gait training with hybrid system (bracing combined with FES) in SCI

High level of energy demand and high effort and loads on the upper limb joints announced the main complication of the orthotics gait rehabilitation with mechanical orthoses. Combination of the mechanical orthoses and FES innovated to improve gait parameters and reduce the loads and energy demand in SCI subjects. The main concept of the using this type of approach announced trunk and hip stability and facilitate forward progression.

Different studies in this field evaluated the hybrid systems on the walking capacity in SCI subjects [38, 40, 48, 49]. Distance walked was announced as 180–1400 m in these studies [38, 40, 48, 49]. Although there was no significant improvement in the walking speed, but improvement in the distance walked was observed in trails in this field. The rate of the distance walked was announced between 3 and 400 m when the FES or orthoses were trained alone [38, 40, 48]. In subjects with incomplete level of spinal cord injury, the gait training with hybrid systems provided improvement in ambulation capacity compared to bracing or FES using alone [50].

9. Orthotic gait training protocol

The training approach announced different among the studies on SCI population [51]. Training protocol has been performed different for powered and mechanical orthoses. Based on the time of the training program, five studies had a shorter training period [26, 45, 52–55], while several weeks to months were reported in other studies [32, 51]. Training protocol was being done on the different surfaces including sidewalk, grass, or stairs [56–58]. Yong et al. used the training protocol with powered gait orthosis on the treadmill to increase confidence of SCI subjects and improvement of the walking speed on them [59]. While in using powered gait orthosis, Arazpour et al. [60] performed upper extremity strengthening and lower extremity stretching as the main section of the training during orthotic gait rehabilitation. Further study on how different training programs affected the walking ability outcomes in the SCI patients will be beneficial in this field.

Orthotic training in SCI subjects can be reduced fatigue and fear of falling and increased the stepping [61]. It was announced that after training program, SCI subjects had walking ability and performance of activity of daily living. The SCI subjects may have less energy demand during walking with orthoses compared to without orthotic gait training condition [32].

10. Positive results of walking in SCI subjects

Complications of SCI such as spasticity, joint contractures, pressure sores, osteoporosis, and urinary tract infections may be present in subjects with SCI [1, 2]. Standing and walking provides physiological and psychological benefits for individuals with SCI [3]. A reduction of bed sores, osteoporosis, spasticity, contractures, and improvement of bladder and bowel functions have all been announced after standing and walking in subjects with SCI [1, 4]. Orthotic gait training is the intervention, which can help in SCI subjects.

Future study in this field must be focused on the following terms:

- The effect of orthotics gait training on the quality of life in SCI subjects

- The effect of orthotics gait training on the electromyography of the lower limb muscles

- Comparison between orthotics gait training with RGOs and powered orthosis on the walking parameters and other related parameters

Author details

Mokhtar Arazpour[1]*, Guive Sharifi[2], Mohammad Ebrahim Mousavi[1] and Maryam Maleki[1]

*Address all correspondence to: m.arazpour@yahoo.com

1 Department of Orthotics and Prosthetics, University of Social Welfare and Rehabilitation Sciences, Tehran, Iran

2 Department of Neurosurgery, Shahid Beheshti University of Medical Sciences, Tehran, Iran

References

[1] Eng JJ, Levins SM, Townson AF, Mah-Jones D, Bremner J, Huston G. Use of prolonged standing for individuals with spinal cord injuries. Physical Therapy. 2001;**81**(8):1392-1399

[2] Anson C, Shepherd C. Incidence of secondary complications in spinal cord injury. International Journal of Rehabilitation Research. 1996;**19**(1):55-66

[3] Walter SJ, Sola GP, Sacks J, Lucero Y, Langbein E, Weaver F. Indications for a home standing program for individuals with spinal cord injury. The Journal of Spinal Cord Medicine. 1999;**22**(3):152-158

[4] Blackmer J. Orthostatic hypotension in spinal cord injured patients. The Journal of Spinal Cord Medicine. 1997;**20**(2):212-217

[5] Ahmadi Bani M, Arazpour M, Farahmand F, Mousavi ME, Hutchins SW. The efficiency of mechanical orthoses in affecting parameters associated with daily living in spinal cord injury patients: A literature review. Disability and Rehabilitation. Assistive Technology. 2015;**10**(3):183-190

[6] Nene A, Hermens H, Zilvold G. Paraplegic locomotion: A review. Spinal Cord. 1996;**34**(9): 507-524

[7] Cheng Y-Y, Hsieh W-L, Kao C-L, Chan R-C. Principles of rehabilitation for common chronic neurologic diseases in the elderly. Journal of Clinical Gerontology and Geriatrics. 2012;**3**(1):5-13

[8] Lovely RG, Gregor R, Roy R, Edgerton V. Effects of training on the recovery of full-weight-bearing stepping in the adult spinal cat. Experimental Neurology. 1986;**92**(2):421-435

[9] Edgerton V, De Leon R, Tillakaratne N, Recktenwald M, Hodgson J, Roy R. Use-dependent plasticity in spinal stepping and standing. Advances in Neurology. 1997;**72**:233-247

[10] De Leon R, Hodgson J, Roy R, Edgerton V. Locomotor capacity attributable to step training versus spontaneous recovery after spinalization in adult cats. Journal of Neurophysiology. 1998;**79**(3):1329-1340

[11] Wirz M, Colombo G, Dietz V. Long term effects of locomotor training in spinal humans. Journal of Neurology, Neurosurgery & Psychiatry. 2001;**71**(1):93-96

[12] Dietz V. Neuronal plasticity after a human spinal cord injury: Positive and negative effects. Experimental Neurology. 2012;**235**(1):110-115

[13] Dietz V. Body weight supported gait training: From laboratory to clinical setting. Brain Research Bulletin. 2009;**78**(1):I-VI

[14] Dietz V, Müller R, Colombo G. Locomotor activity in spinal man: Significance of afferent input from joint and load receptors. Brain. 2002;**125**(12):2626-2634

[15] Lam T, Eng J, Wolfe D, Hsieh J, Whittaker M. A systematic review of the efficacy of gait rehabilitation strategies for spinal cord injury. Topics in Spinal Cord Injury Rehabilitation. 2007;**13**(1):32-57

[16] Barbeau H, Fung J. The role of rehabilitation in the recovery of walking in the neurological population. Current Opinion in Neurology. 2001;**14**(6):735-740

[17] Ferris D, Sawicki G, Domingo A. Powered lower limb orthoses for gait rehabilitation. Topics in Spinal Cord Injury Rehabilitation. 2005;**11**(2):34-49

[18] Colombo G, Schreier R, Mayr A, Plewa H, Rupp R. Novel tilt table with integrated robotic stepping mechanism: Design principles and clinical application. In: Proc. IEEE 9th Int. Conf. Rehabilitation Robotics. 2005, p. 227-230

[19] Chi L, Masani K, Miyatani M, Thrasher TA, Johnston KW, Mardimae A, et al. Cardiovascular response to functional electrical stimulation and dynamic tilt table therapy to improve orthostatic tolerance. Journal of Electromyography and Kinesiology. 2008;**18**(6):900-907

[20] Czell D, Schreier R, Rupp R, Eberhard S, Colombo G, Dietz V. Influence of passive leg movements on blood circulation on the tilt table in healthy adults. Journal of Neuroengineering and Rehabilitation. 2004;**1**(1):4

[21] Li W, Huang Y, Xu J, Jiping H. Brain activity during walking in patient with spinal cord injury. 2011 International Symposium on Bioelectronics and Bioinformatics (ISBB). 2011, p. 96-99

[22] Laubacher M, Perret C, Hunt KJ. Work-rate-guided exercise testing in patients with incomplete spinal cord injury using a robotics-assisted tilt-table. Disability and Rehabilitation. Assistive Technology. 2015;**10**(5):433-438

[23] Yoshida T, Masani K, Sayenko DG, Miyatani M, Fisher JA, Popovic MR. Cardiovascular response of individuals with spinal cord injury to dynamic functional electrical stimulation under orthostatic stress. IEEE Transactions on Neural Systems and Rehabilitation Engineering. 2013;**21**(1):37-46

[24] Herrero A, Menendez H, Gil L, Martin J, Martin T, Garcia-Lopez D, et al. Effects of whole-body vibration on blood flow and neuromuscular activity in spinal cord injury. Spinal Cord. 2011;**49**(4):554

[25] Liu DS, Chang WH, Wong AM, Chen S-C, Lin K-P, Lai C-H. Development of a biofeedback tilt-table for investigating orthostatic syncope in patients with spinal cord injury. Medical and Biological Engineering and Computing. 2007;**45**(12):1223-1228

[26] Evans N, Hartigan C, Kandilakis C, Pharo E, Clesson I. Acute cardiorespiratory and metabolic responses during exoskeleton-assisted walking overground among persons with chronic spinal cord injury. Topics in Spinal Cord Injury Rehabilitation. 2015;**21**(2):122-132

[27] Thrasher TA, Keller T, Lawrence M, Popovic MR. Effects of isometric FES and dynamic FES on cardiovascular parameters on an active tilt-table stepper. In: Proc. 10th Int. Funct. Electr. Stimulat. Soc. Conf. 2005, p. 409-411

[28] Hornby TG, Zemon DH, Campbell D. Robotic-assisted, body-weight–supported treadmill training in individuals following motor incomplete spinal cord injury. Physical Therapy. 2005;**85**(1):52-66

[29] Hornby TG, Reinkensmeyer DJ, Chen D. Manually-assisted versus robotic-assisted body weight-supported treadmill training in spinal cord injury: What is the role of each? PM&R. 2010;**2**(3):214-221

[30] Arazpour M, Bani MA, Hutchins SW. Reciprocal gait orthoses and powered gait orthoses for walking by spinal cord injury patients. Prosthetics and Orthotics International. 2013;**37**(1):14-21

[31] Ahmadi Bani M, Arazpour M, Farahmand F, Mousavi ME, Hutchins SW. The efficiency of mechanical orthoses in affecting parameters associated with daily living in spinal cord injury patients: A literature review. Disability and Rehabilitation. Assistive Technology. 2014;(0):1-8

[32] Samadian M, Arazpour M, Bani MA, Pouyan A, Bahramizadeh M, Hutchins S. The influence of orthotic gait training with an isocentric reciprocating gait orthosis on the walking ability of paraplegic patients: A pilot study. Spinal Cord. 2015

[33] Harvey LA, Davis GM, Smith MB, Engel S. Energy expenditure during gait using the walkabout and isocentric reciprocal gait orthoses in persons with paraplegia. Archives of Physical Medicine and Rehabilitation. 1998;**79**(8):945-949

[34] Harvey LA, Smith MB, Davis GM, Engel S. Functional outcomes attained by T9-12 paraplegic patients with the walkabout and the isocentric reciprocal gait orthoses. Archives of Physical Medicine and Rehabilitation. 1997;**78**(7):706-711

[35] Harvey LA, Newton-John T, Davis GM, Smith MB, Engel S. A comparison of the attitude of paraplegic individuals to the walkabout orthosis and the isocentric reciprocal gait orthosis. Spinal Cord. 1997;**35**(9):580-584

[36] Onogi K, Kondo I, Saitoh E, Kato M, Oyobe T. Comparison of the effects of sliding-type and hinge-type joints of knee-ankle-foot orthoses on temporal gait parameters in patients with paraplegia. Japanese Journal of Comprehensive Rehabilitation Science. 2010;**1**:1-6

[37] Robinett CS, Vondran MA. Functional ambulation velocity and distance requirements in rural and urban communities: A clinical report. Physical Therapy. 1988;**68**(9):1371-1373

[38] Sykes L, Edwards J, Powell ES, Ross ERS. The reciprocating gait orthosis: Long-term usage patterns. Archives of Physical Medicine and Rehabilitation. 1995;**76**(8):779-783

[39] Hong C, San Luis E, Chung S. Follow-up study on the use of leg braces issued to spinal cord injury patients. Spinal Cord. 1990;**28**(3):172-177

[40] Thoumie P, Perrouin-Verbe B, Le Claire G, Bedoiseau M, Busnel M, Cormerais A, et al. Restoration of functional gait in paraplegic patients with the RGO-II hybrid orthosis. A multicentre controlled study. I. Clinical evaluation. Spinal Cord. 1995;**33**(11):647-653

[41] Franceschini M, Baratta S, Zampolini M, Loria D, Lotta S. Reciprocating gait orthoses: A multicenter study of their use by spinal cord injured patients. Archives of Physical Medicine and Rehabilitation. 1997;**78**(6):582-586

[42] Suzuki K, Mito G, Kawamoto H, Hasegawa Y, Sankai Y. Intention-based walking support for paraplegia patients with robot suit HAL. Advanced Robotics. 2007;**21**(12):1441-1469

[43] Middleton JW, Sinclair PJ, Smith RM, Davis GM. Postural control during stance in paraplegia: Effects of medially linked versus unlinked knee-ankle-foot orthoses. Archives of Physical Medicine and Rehabilitation. 1999;**80**(12):1558-1565

[44] Tsukahara A, Hasegawa Y, Sankai Y. Gait support for complete spinal cord injury patient by synchronized leg-swing with HAL. 2011 IEEE/RSJ International Conference on Intelligent Robots and Systems (IROS)

[45] Zeilig G, Weingarden H, Zwecker M, Dudkiewicz I, Bloch A, Esquenazi A. Safety and tolerance of the ReWalk™ exoskeleton suit for ambulation by people with complete spinal cord injury: A pilot study. The Journal of Spinal Cord Medicine. 2012;**35**(2):96-101

[46] Esquenazi A, Talaty M, Packel A, Saulino M. The ReWalk powered exoskeleton to restore ambulatory function to individuals with thoracic-level motor-complete spinal cord injury. American Journal of Physical Medicine & Rehabilitation. 2012;**91**(11):911-921

[47] Tanabe S, Saitoh E, Hirano S, Katoh M, Takemitsu T, Uno A, et al. Design of the wearable power-assist locomotor (WPAL) for paraplegic gait reconstruction. Disability and Rehabilitation. Assistive Technology. 2013;**8**(1):84-91

[48] Marsolais E, Kobetic R, Polando G, Ferguson K, Tashman S, Gaudio R, et al. The Case Western Reserve University hybrid gait orthosis. The Journal of Spinal Cord Medicine. 1999;**23**(2):100-108

[49] Solomonow M, et al. FES powered locomotion of paraplegics fitted with the LSU reciprocating gait orthoses (RGO). In: Proc. Annual Int. Con6 IEEE Eng. Medicine and Biology Soc. 1988;**10**:1672

[50] Kim CM, Eng JJ, Whittaker MW. Effects of a simple functional electric system and/or a hinged ankle-foot orthosis on walking in persons with incomplete spinal cord injury. Archives of Physical Medicine and Rehabilitation. 2004;**85**(10):1718-1723

[51] Louie DR, Eng JJ, Lam T. Gait speed using powered robotic exoskeletons after spinal cord injury: A systematic review and correlational study. Journal of Neuroengineering and Rehabilitation. 2015;**12**(1):1

[52] Hartigan C, Kandilakis C, Dalley S, Clausen M, Wilson E, Morrison S, et al. Mobility outcomes following five training sessions with a powered exoskeleton. Topics in Spinal Cord Injury Rehabilitation. 2015;**21**(2):93-99

[53] Kolakowsky-Hayner SA, Crew J, Moran S, Shah A. Safety and feasibility of using the EksoTM bionic exoskeleton to aid ambulation after spinal cord injury. Journal of Spine. 2013;**2013**

[54] Neuhaus PD, Noorden JH, Craig TJ, Torres T, Kirschbaum J, Pratt JE. Design and evaluation of mina: A robotic orthosis for paraplegics. Paper presented at the IEEE International Conference on Rehabilitation Robotics: ICORR 2011, Zurich, CH. (2011, Jun 29–Jul 1)

[55] Tanabe S, Hirano S, Saitoh E. Wearable power-assist Locomotor (WPAL) for supporting upright walking in persons with paraplegia. NeuroRehabilitation. 2013;**33**(1):99-106

[56] Kozlowski A, Bryce T, Dijkers M. Time and effort required by persons with spinal cord injury to learn to use a powered exoskeleton for assisted walking. Topics in Spinal Cord Injury Rehabilitation. 2015;**21**(2):110-121

[57] Fineberg DB, Asselin P, Harel NY, Agranova-Breyter I, Kornfeld SD, Bauman WA, et al. Vertical ground reaction force-based analysis of powered exoskeleton-assisted walking in persons with motor-complete paraplegia. The Journal of Spinal Cord Medicine. 2013;**36**(4):313-321

[58] Benson I, Hart K, Tussler D, van Middendorp JJ. Lower-limb exoskeletons for individuals with chronic spinal cord injury: Findings from a feasibility study. Clin Rehabil. 2016 Jan;**30**(1):73-84

[59] Yang A, Asselin P, Knezevic S, Kornfeld S, Spungen A. Assessment of in-hospital walking velocity and level of assistance in a powered exoskeleton in persons with spinal cord injury. Topics in Spinal Cord Injury Rehabilitation. 2015;**21**(2):100-109

[60] Arazpour M, Bani M, Hutchins S, Jones R. The physiological cost index of walking with mechanical and powered gait orthosis in patients with spinal cord injury. Spinal Cord. 2013;**51**(5):356-359

[61] Arazpour M, Bani M, Hutchins S, Curran S, Javanshir M. The influence of ankle joint mobility when using an orthosis on stability in patients with spinal cord injury: A pilot study. Spinal Cord. 2013;**51**(10):750

2

Docosahexaenoic Acid Promotes Recovery of Motor Function by Neuroprotection and Neuroplasticity Mechanisms

John V. Priestley and Adina T. Michael-Titus

Abstract

The omega-3 polyunsaturated fatty acid, docosahexaenoic acid (DHA), has been shown to promote recovery of motor function after spinal cord injury. This is likely to be at least partly due to neuroprotective effects of DHA. However, recent studies have shown that DHA also supports neuroplasticity after injury, such as promoting sprouting of spared corticospinal tract (CST) axons. In this chapter, we review the published studies showing that DHA promotes recovery of motor function in rodent models of spinal cord injury (SCI), and consider the available data on the underlying mechanisms. This includes effects on inflammation and on neuronal and oligodendrocyte survival at the injury site, and effects on spared CST axons and serotonergic axons. Current data support the hypothesis that DHA promotes recovery of motor function by both neuroprotection and neuroplasticity mechanisms. The significance of this, and the implications of combining DHA with rehabilitation strategies, will be discussed.

Keywords: thoracic spinal cord injury, cervical spinal cord injury, central pattern generator, V2a interneurons, DHA

1. Introduction

1.1. Polyunsaturated fatty acids and their role in neurology

Polyunsaturated fatty acids (PUFA) of the omega-3 and omega-6 series are lipids with major structural and signalling roles. The long-chain omega-3 PUFA docosahexaenoic acid (DHA) is present in significant concentrations in the central nervous system (CNS), where its synthesis from the dietary precursor alpha-linolenic acid (LNA) occurs through desaturation, elongation and β-oxidation reactions. Its intermediate precursors are eicosapentaenoic acid (EPA) and docosapentaenoic acid (DPA). In humans, the conversion of LNA into DHA is below 5% [1, 2]. Therefore, an adequate dietary supply of DHA is required, especially because due to modern food manufacturing, there has been a significant decrease in the omega-3 intake and the omega-3 to omega-6 PUFA dietary ratio in the Western diet [3]. These changes have been linked to an increase in the incidence and the prevalence of diseases such as cancer, cardiovascular disease, rheumatoid arthritis, osteoporosis and asthma [4]. After absorption, the omega-3 PUFA can cross cellular membranes through specialized fatty acid transporters and interact with fatty acid-binding proteins (FABP). These proteins are a family of lipid chaperones involved in the extracellular and intracellular transport of fatty acids [5]. FABP bind long-chain fatty acids, with different ligand selectivity and binding affinity profiles. Changes in FABP levels have been reported following injury. For example, B-FABP is found in the brain and has very high affinity for DHA; it is detected in plasma as a high specificity and sensitivity biomarker of brain injury [6]. More recently, Figueroa et al. [7] reported increases in tissue levels of FABP-5 after spinal cord injury.

The principal omega-3 PUFA in the brain is DHA, representing 10–20% of the total fatty acid composition. Retinal tissue is also highly enriched in DHA. This fatty acid is a component of phospholipids, in particular phosphatidylethanolamine and phosphatidylserine; it is concentrated in cytoplasmic and synaptosomal membranes, growth cones, microsomal and mitochondrial membranes, and is also a component of myelin [8]. DHA-enriched phospholipids are present in the inner leaflet of the cytoplasmic membrane, and DHA chains are very flexible and transition rapidly between conformational states. This creates a unique microenvironment for the functioning of many proteins embedded in membranes, such as neurotransmitter receptors [9]. After release from membrane phospholipids by phospholipases, long-chain omega-3 PUFA such as DHA can be metabolized and produce a wide range of metabolites, designated with the generic term of "docosanoids", which include protectins, D-series resolvins and maresins. These DHA metabolites have intrinsic biological effects, which are mediated through specific receptors [10, 11]. Therefore, some of the effects induced by DHA may be due not to a direct action of the fatty acid but to specific metabolites which are derived from it, and which could attain significant levels, especially under conditions of chronic DHA supplementation [12].

DHA has an essential role in normal neurodevelopment, in particular for vision and cognition [13]. Supplementation with DHA has been shown to improve various aspects of learning and memory in children [14]. More than two decades ago, Martinez and collaborators [15] carried out seminal studies in children with peroxysomal disorders, which lead to a major DHA deficit, and showed that supplementation with DHA can lead to significant improvement in neurological function, and this is accompanied by improved myelination of the immature brain. At around the same time, studies initiated by Lazdunski and collaborators were providing evidence that omega-3 PUFA had significant neuroprotective potential under conditions which lead to CNS injury, such as seizures and ischaemia [16]. DHA has been increasingly linked to a variety of conditions, such as Alzheimer's disease and Parkinson's disease, and also schizophrenia, depression and attention deficit-hyperactivity disorder [17–19], and this has consolidated the idea that dietary supplementation with DHA could have therapeutic value across a spectrum of major disorders in neurology and psychiatry.

1.2. Pathways controlling movement in the rat and possible strategies for promoting recovery of movement following spinal cord injury (SCI)

Locomotion in rodents is controlled by a central pattern generator (CPG) which generates the basic rhythm of limb flexion and extension and which, for the hindlimbs, is located in the lower thoracic and upper lumbar spinal cord. In recent years, great progress has been made in dissecting the organization of the CPG, by identifying subtypes of neurons based on their developmental expression of specific transcription factors (summarized in [20, 21]). Genetic ablation of specific transcription factors can then be used to probe the functional roles of different neuronal subtypes (see e.g. [22, 23]). **Figure 1** illustrates one possible model of the

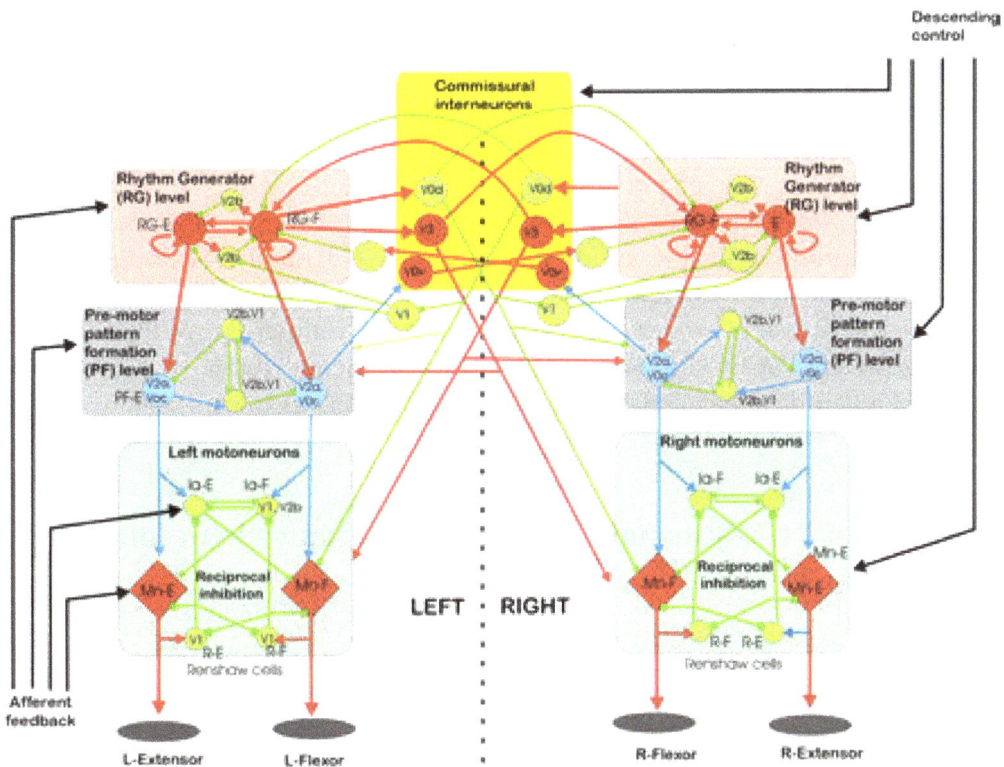

Figure 1. Schematic model of the rodent CPG controlling hind limb movement. Excitatory neurons are shown in red, and inhibitory neurons are shown in green. Rhythm generator (RG), pattern formation (PF) and motoneurons (Mn) are present for both flexion and extension on both sides of the spinal cord. V0d, V0v, V0c, V1, V2a, V2b and V3 are different types of interneurons which in some cases correspond to existing well-characterized neuronal types (e.g. V1 neurons include Renshaw cells). V2a neurons are shown in blue and have direct projections to motoneurons, plus projections to V2b/V1 PF inhibitory interneurons and to V0v excitatory commissural interneurons. Afferent feedback and descending control occur bilaterally, but for simplicity have only been shown ipsilaterally. The diagram is based on diagrams contained in Harris-Warrick [20] and Rybak and colleagues [21].

CPG based on studies reported in [22, 23]. Flexor and extensor motoneurons are thought to have separate rhythm generators (RG) which provide input to a pattern formation (PF) network that controls flexor/extensor alternation. The RG network also connects to commissural interneurons which coordinate left/right hindlimb movement. As an example of the complexity of the system, we have highlighted the V2a class of excitatory interneuron in **Figure 1**. V2a neurons can be identified by their expression of the homeodomain protein Chx10 and receive input from the RG centres. They project to three different targets, namely (1) motoneurons, (2) V2b inhibitory interneurons that are part of the PF centre, and (3) V0v commissural interneurons [21]. They therefore can influence locomotion by direct monosynaptic inputs to motoneurons and by regulating the flexor/extensor and left/right coordinating centres. However, V2a interneurons are not only present in the lumbar CPG, they also occur in the cervical spinal cord and play a key role in skilled forelimb movement, by conveying an internal copy of the premotor signals. This is possible because of their dual innervation of cervical motoneurons and precerebellar interneurons [22].

The CPG can generate alternating hindlimb movements independently, but in the intact animal, the CPG is modulated by afferent feedback and by descending control. The effects of SCI depend on the spinal level of the injury. Rats subject to complete transection above the level of the lumbar locomotor centres show some spontaneous recovery of hindlimb movement [24], and this can be increased by a variety of treatments, including weight supported treadmill training [24], delivery of growth factors [25, 26] and implantation of various exogenous cells [27–29]. At least some of this recovery of function appears to be related to regeneration or sprouting of descending bulbospinal [30, 31] and corticospinal [25] pathways. In contrast, the lasting paraplegia that results from a SCI at lumbar level is thought to result from loss of spinal interneurons, possibly including components of the CPG [32]. An efficacious treatment for SCI might need to preserve and/or restore descending control pathways and repair damage to intrinsic networks such as the CPG.

2. The effects of PUFA treatment on recovery of movement following experimental SCI

2.1. Thoracic hemisection SCI

DHA promotes recovery of quadrupedal locomotion in rats and mice following thoracic hemisection [33], compression [34–36] and contusion [37] SCI, when acutely administered post-injury. Recovery is further improved if an acute injection of DHA is followed by a DHA-supplemented diet (**Figure 2**). The DHA treatment results in increased neuronal and oligodendrocyte survival [34] and decreased macrophage and microglial activation [36, 38] at the injury site. However, since the motoneuron pools that contribute to locomotion are not at thoracic level, it is likely that the effects on locomotion are due to preservation of descending axons passing through the injury site rather than preservation of thoracic neurons themselves. Analysis of axon numbers at the SCI site using generic axonal markers such as neurofilament and myelin basic protein (MBP) reveals that DHA preserves axons in white matter tracts [39] but, with the exception of serotonin (5-hydroxytryptamine, 5-HT), the origin and role of those axons have not been much explored. As outlined above, corticospinal and bulbospinal projections play an important role in motor control but mainly innervate moto-neurons indirectly, via interneurons, and so are difficult to analyse (however, see Section 4 on pyramidotomy below). In contrast, 5-HT axons are derived from the medullary raphe nuclei, innervate many motoneurons monosynaptically and play key roles in modulating motoneur-on excitability [40]. DHA treatment preserves the number of 5-HT axons at the level of a thoracic compression injury [39], including axons that appear to contact motoneurons (see **Figure 3**). It is therefore likely that at least some of the motor recovery is due to increased preservation of 5-HT axons that pass through the injury site and innervate motoneurons at lumbar level. 5-HT axons have a great capacity to sprout and make new connections [41]. Another possibility is therefore that some 5-HT axons are spared by the SCI but that DHA promotes sprouting and restoration of synaptic circuits by these axons. These possibilities have not been examined directly following thoracic SCI, but the effects of DHA on 5-HT axons have been studied in much more detail following cervical injury.

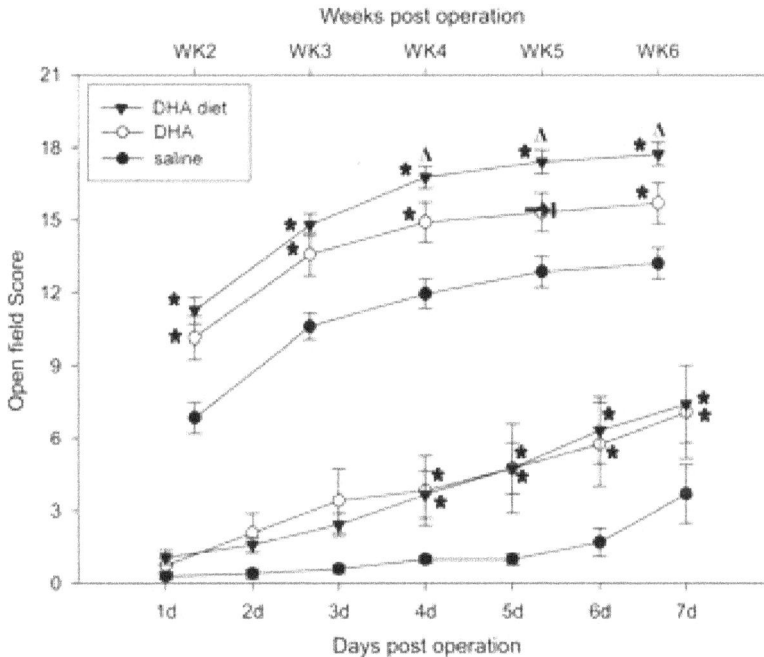

Figure 2. Locomotor performance of thoracic compression SCI rats injected with saline or DHA and of animals injected with DHA and then fed on a DHA-enriched diet. Results for days 1–7 are shown in the bottom half of the graph, plotted against the bottom X-axis. Results for 2–6 weeks are shown in the top half of the graph, plotted against the top X-axis. Both DHA- and saline-treated animals showed similar low levels of locomotor function 1 day after surgery, as assessed on the BBB open field task. During the first week, DHA-treated animals had improved motor function recovery compared with saline-treated animals (days 5, 6 and 7; $*p < 0.05$). Between week 2 and week 6, DHA-treated animals continued to perform better than saline-treated animals ($*p < 0.05$). In addition, from the 4th week onwards, animals injected with DHA followed by maintenance on the DHA-enriched diet, performed better than animals only injected with DHA (weeks 4, 5 and 6; $^\Delta p < 0.05$). Error bars represent SEMs. Reproduced from [34] with permission.

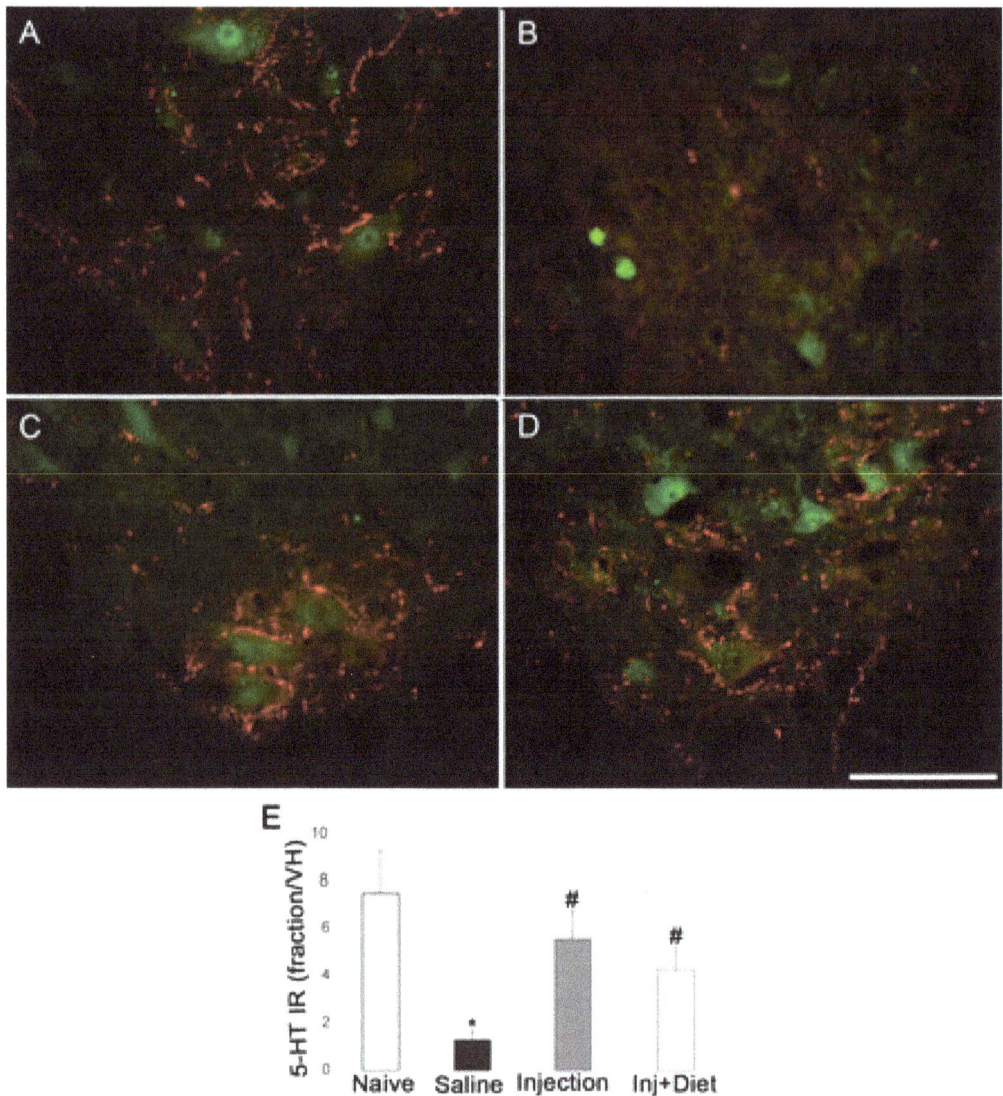

Figure 3. Immunofluorescence micrographs showing thin, 5-HT immunoreactive (IR) axons (red) that innervate NeuN labelled neurons (green) in the ventral horn (VH). In naïve animals (A), a dense network of beaded 5-HT-positive fibres can be seen surrounding large NeuN neurons. At 6 weeks post-thoracic compression injury, a marked loss of 5-HT-positive fibres was seen in saline-treated animals (B) compared with the groups receiving DHA injection alone (C), or in combination with a DHA-enriched diet (D). Quantitative analysis (E) at 6 weeks post-injury revealed a significant loss of 5-HT IR in the VH of saline-treated animals following injury. A significant amelioration in the loss of 5-HT IR was observed in the VH in both DHA-treatment groups (significantly different from *naïve or #saline-treated animals at $p < 0.05$; scale bar = 100 μm). Reproduced from [39] with permission.

2.2. Experimental cervical SCI

The majority of experimental studies have focused on thoracic injury, but the most common clinical injury is at cervical level (57% of SCI). Recently, we have therefore examined the effects of DHA in a cervical (C5 level) hemisection SCI model [42]. The cervical level of injury also has the advantage of allowing us to examine the effects of DHA treatment on a skilled motor task, namely retrieval of food using the forepaws. Rats are trained to retrieve food by extending a forelimb through a gap in a perspex box and grasping food pellets which are on a staircase [43]. Following SCI at C5 level, rats lose the ability to recover the food pellets, but recover partial function if treated acutely with DHA (**Figure 4**). Following cervical hemisection, 5-HT axons show a remarkable degree of plasticity. Rostral to the hemisection, there is an increase in 5-HT immunoreactivity which is maintained up to 3 weeks. Caudal to the hemisection, there is a transient loss of 5-HT immunoreactivity at 1 week, but levels are restored by 3 weeks (**Figure 5B**). DHA treatment results in an even greater number of 5-HT immunoreactive axons caudal to the injury (**Figure 5B**), and increased density of 5-HT axons contacting motoneurons (**Figure 5C–E**). However, 5-HT axons are not the only ones to sprout in response to DHA treatment. Corticospinal tract (CST) axons on the intact side of the spinal cord were identified by anterograde labelling with the tracer biotinylated dextran amine (BDA). Following hemisection, a small number of these axons sprout across the midline to innervate the denervated side of the spinal cord. However, after DHA treatment, this number doubles [42]. It is therefore possible that the recovery of skilled movement is due to sprouting of 5-HT and CST axons and formation of novel circuits. However, since the increase in axons occurs at the same level as the hemisection, it is possible that the increase in 5-HT and CST axons is due to neuroprotection rather than neuroplasticity. We have therefore examined the effect of DHA treatment in a third model of SCI, namely unilateral pyramidotomy in the mouse [42].

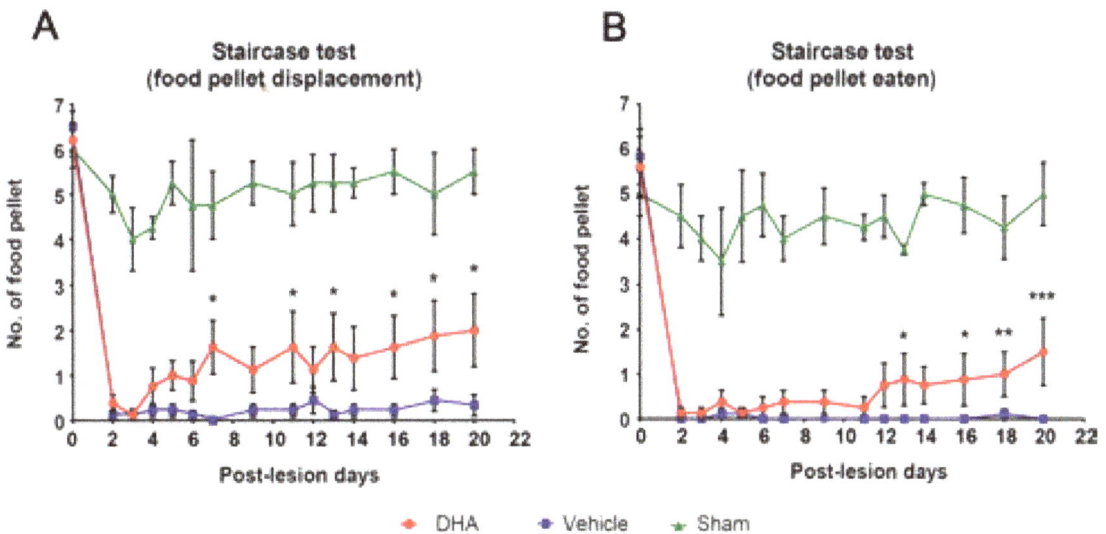

Figure 4. DHA enhances functional recovery following cervical lateral hemisection in the rat. A, B, In the Montoya staircase test, all injured animals lost the ability to displace (gross motor function) or eat (fine motor function) the food pellet after cervical lateral hemisection 2 d after injury. The animals treated with vehicle did not recover any food retrieval ability (blue squares), but DHA-treated animals gradually recovered food retrieval ability (red circles) from around 2 weeks onwards, compared with uninjured sham operated animals (green triangles). *$p < 0.05$, **$p < 0.01$, ***$p < 0.001$, compared to vehicle-treated animals. Results represent mean ± SEM. Reproduced from [42] with permission.

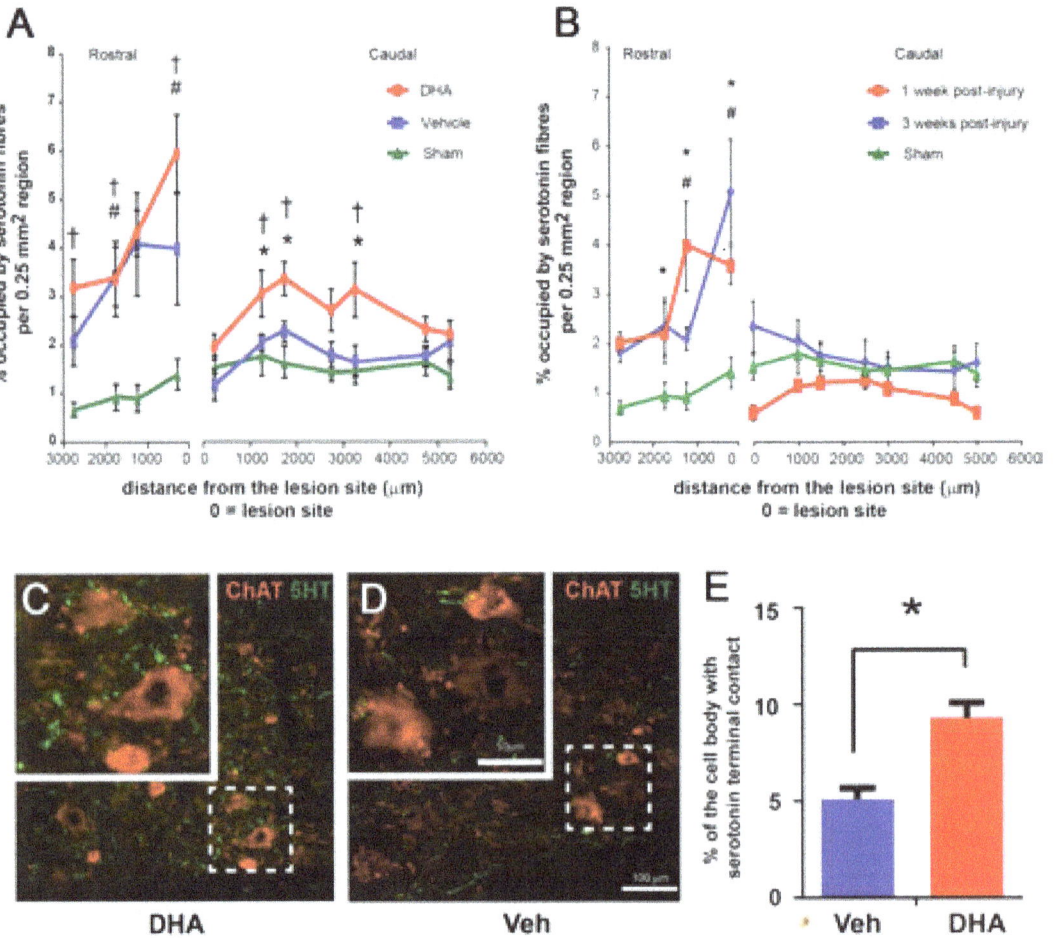

Figure 5. DHA enhances 5-HT (serotonin) fibre regrowth following cervical lateral hemisection in the rat. (*A*) Serotonin fibres in the rostral part of the lesion site were significantly increased in both treatment groups at 3 weeks post-injury, but only the DHA-treated group (red circles), not the vehicle group (blue squares), had significantly increased serotonin in the caudal region compared with the sham operated animals (green triangles). (*B*) Serotonin fibres in the rostral part of the lesion site were significantly increased at 1 week (red square) and 3 weeks (blue circle) compared with the sham operated group after lateral cervical hemisection. However, in the caudal region, 1 and 3 weeks after injury were similar to the sham operated group. 1 week after hemisection, there was a loss of serotonin but by 3 weeks levels had returned to values similar to sham operated animals. $N = 5$ or 6 per group. #$p < 0.05$, 1 week hemisection versus sham group. *$p < 0.05$, 3 week hemisection versus sham group. (*C*, *D*) The images were captured 1750 μm caudal to the lesion site. Double labelling shows serotonin fibres (green) in contact with ChAT immunoreactive motor neurons (red) in the ventral horn of vehicle- and DHA-treated rats. Insets, dashed boxes at higher magnification. (*E*) Quantitative analysis reveals that there is a significant increase in the density of serotonin fibres contacting motor neurons in the DHA-treated group compared with the control group. $N = 5$ or 6 per group. *$p < 0.05$, DHA versus vehicle group. †$p < 0.05$, sham versus vehicle group. #$p < 0.05$, DHA versus sham group. Scale bar, 100 μm. Reproduced from [42] with permission.

2.3. Pyramidotomy

The CST axons in rodents run in the medullary pyramids, before decussating and descending at the base of the dorsal columns. Unilateral pyramidotomy transects these CST axons and

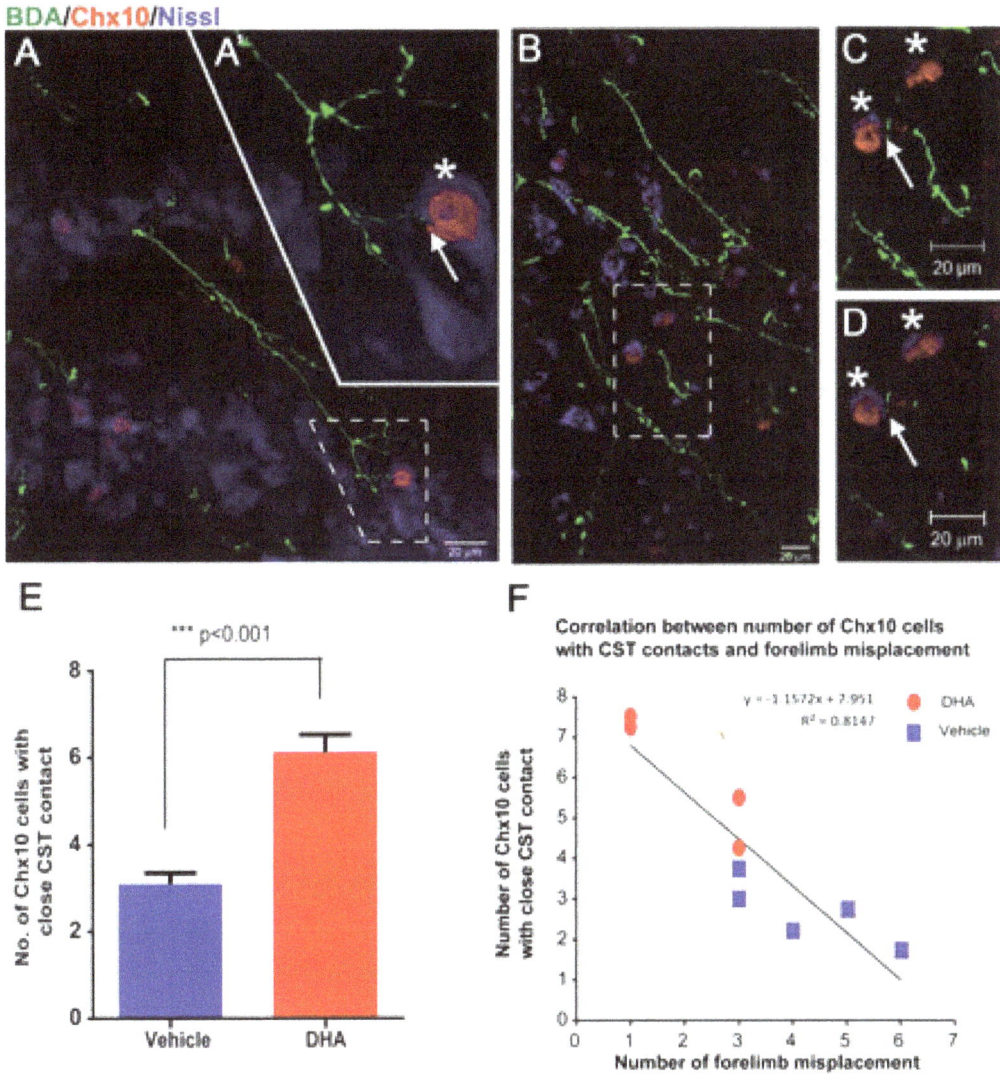

Figure 6. DHA enhances functional recovery via connection with Chx10 interneurons in pyramidotomy mice. (*A–D*), Confocal images of mouse cervical spinal cord transverse sections at the intermediate laminae of the CST-denervated side, showing examples of BDA-labelled CST collaterals (green) in the vicinity of blue fluorescent Nissl-stained cells (Neurotrace 435/455), some of which are V2a interneurons identified by immunostaining for Chx10 (red). (*A, B*) Dashed boxes represent high magnification in *A'*, and in *C, D*, which reveal contacts (arrows) between BDA-labelled collaterals and Chx10 interneurons (asterisks). (*A'*) A Z-stack comprising 10 × 0.66 μm optical images. (*C*), A stack comprising 25 × 0.72 μm optical images. (*D, A*) Single 0.72 μm optical image. Examination of the single optical image confirms that the BDA-labelled CST fibre contacts (arrow) one of the Chx10 interneurons. (*E*) Quantitative analysis revealed a significant increase in the number of Chx10 interneurons contacted by BDA-labelled CST collaterals following DHA treatment (red bar) compared with vehicle treatment (blue bar). (*F*) A strong negative correlation was observed between the numbers of Chx10 interneurons with BDA-labelled CST contacts and the numbers of forelimb misplacements. Data were taken from DHA-treated (red circle) and vehicle-treated (blue square) animals. ***$p<0.001$, DHA versus vehicle group. Scale bar, 20 μm. Reproduced from [42] with permission.

results in the loss of CST axons in the spinal cord on the contralateral side. Using BDA to label the CST axons on the non-lesioned side, we observed that a small number of CST axons respond to the pyramidotomy by sprouting across the midline to innervate the lesioned side (**Figure 6A**). The number of sprouting CST axons is doubled following DHA treatment [42]. Furthermore, we have shown that the sprouting axons contact a particular class of interneuron, namely the V2a propriospinal neurons described above. V2a neurons were identified by their expression of the Chx10 transcription factor (**Figure 6A–D**). V2a interneurons have been shown to play an important role in skilled reaching [22]. Following DHA treatment and pyramidotomy, an increased number of V2a interneurons receive contacts from CST axons (**Figure 6E**), and the recovery of forelimb movement shows a tight correlation with the number of V2a neurons that receive contacts (**Figure 6F**). It therefore appears that DHA treatment after pyramidotomy results in the formation of a novel circuit (CST to contralateral V2a interneurons) that promotes recovery of skilled reaching. This is in addition to the effects of DHA on sprouting 5-HT axons, and neuroprotective effects on neuronal cell bodies and axons.

3. Discussion

Motor pathways are so complex that it is difficult to establish a direct causal relationship between the effects of a therapeutic agent on spinal circuitry and an improvement in a particular motor task. However, the data reviewed above indicates that there is a strong correlation between the neuroprotective and neuroplasticity effects of DHA and the recovery of motor function. This dual effect of DHA, together with its established safety profile and the recent demonstration of the efficacy in SCI of a multinutrient combination containing DHA and EPA [44], makes DHA a particularly promising candidate for development as a therapeutic agent in SCI. There is a substantial literature on the neuroprotective effects of DHA (reviewed above) but the effects on neuroplasticity are more novel and less studied. We have shown that DHA treatment following SCI upregulates the microRNA miR-21 and suppresses phosphatase and tensin homolog (PTEN), a central negative regulator of the phosphatidylinositol 3-kinase (PI3K) signalling pathway [42]. However, these effects are quite widespread and it is not known how they result in beneficial axon sprouting. Bareyre and colleagues [45] have shown that new connections form after SCI, but inappropriate connections are lost because they are not used. A similar mechanism may mould the sprouting and connections promoted by DHA, in which case, there may be great benefit in combining DHA treatment with rehabilitation and task specific training.

3.1. Therapeutic implications

The magnitude of the effects induced by the acute administration of DHA and reported in various models of SCI is comparable with that described with various other therapeutic approaches which are already being explored in clinical trials in neurotrauma, such as progesterone, erythropoietin, riluzole and minocycline [46]. DHA has clear potential for clinical translation in SCI; therefore, it is appropriate to consider the issues which remain to be clarified in order to improve the chances of translational success.

It is important to note that in the studies published so far with DHA and reporting beneficial effects of this fatty acid in a variety of conditions, there are two types of administration: DHA administered using a chronic oral supplementation route and DHA administered as an acute bolus, using an injectable route. Are the cellular targets and mechanisms activated by DHA the same in the two types of treatment? When DHA is administered chronically, one of the consequences of this regime is the structural enrichment in DHA in membranes, and because DHA has unique molecular structural characteristics, this influences the dynamics of membrane components, and may change the activity of ion channels and G-protein-coupled receptors (GPCR). DHA incorporation in membranes changes the properties of specialized domains such as the lipid rafts and caveolae, and this can modify signalling [47]. When DHA is administered acutely as a bolus, its half-life in plasma is very short (approximately 2 min), as shown in PET imaging studies carried out in healthy volunteers [48]; therefore, efficacy may be due to the activation of different mechanisms. Long-chain omega-3 PUFA such as DHA and EPA have various specific molecular targets, including ion channels, GPCR and nuclear receptors [17, 47]. They include voltage-sensitive Na^+ and Ca^{2+} channels and two-pore domain background K^+ channels, such as TREK-1 (which is also a target for riluzole), the GPCRs GPR40 and GPR120, and transcription factors such as the retinoid X receptors (RXR) and peroxisome proliferator-activated receptors (PPAR). RXR can heterodimerize with PPAR or with retinoic acid receptors (RAR), and changes in the expression of these receptors have been reported after SCI [49]. Several studies indicate that the activation of retinoid signalling supports axonal regeneration [50].

The spontaneous partial recovery of function which occurs after SCI may be due to neuroplasticity, compensation and repair [51]. Rehabilitation through training is at present the most successful treatment for patients with SCI, to enhance the recovery of some neurological function. Rehabilitation enhances the spontaneous plasticity changes that occur after injury and enhances the activity of sensorimotor pathways, as documented in experimental SCI [52]. Exercise leads to a reconfiguration of cortical representation maps, it modifies the biophysical properties of motoneuron membranes, changes the activity of spinal inhibitory circuits and also increases the levels of neurotrophic factors, such as brain-derived neurotrophic factor (BDNF) and neurotrophin-3 (NT-3) [53]. Liu and collaborators [54] have shown that exercise increases the expression of miR21 and decreases PTEN mRNA levels, a profile of effects similar to our observations with DHA. Considering this similarity of action, a goal of future studies should be the exploration of a combination of DHA and exercise, to establish whether what could be achieved is true synergism or only additivity. The concept of combining treatment with exercise is supported by examples such as the successful combination of exercise with strategies such as the reduction in the glial scar components using chondroitinase ABC [55]. However, not all combinations achieve an optimum effect, as shown by the negative results obtained by combining exercise with antibodies against the myelin-derived inhibitor Nogo A [56]. Therefore, it will be essential to continue to characterize the targets and mode of action of DHA, so that it becomes clear what mechanisms could be harnessed and amplified by combining DHA (acute administration and chronic exposure) and rehabilitation training, to optimize outcome in SCI patients.

Acknowledgements

We acknowledge the generous support of Spinal Research, Corporate Action Trust, Barts Charity and Chang Gung Memorial Hospital (Taiwan) for the DHA studies in the various models of SCI discussed here.

Author details

John V. Priestley* and Adina T. Michael-Titus

*Address all correspondence to: j.v.priestley@qmul.ac.uk

Centre for Neuroscience and Trauma, Blizard Institute, Barts and The London School of Medicine and Dentistry, Queen Mary University of London, London, UK

References

[1] BrennaJT, SalemNJr., SinclairAJ, CunnaneSC. alpha-Linolenic acid supplementation and conversion to n-3 long-chain polyunsaturated fatty acids in humans. Prostaglandins Leukot Essent Fatty Acids. 2009; 80: 85–91.

[2] BrennaJT. Efficiency of conversion of alpha-linolenic acid to long chain n-3 fatty acids in man. Curr Opin Clin Nutr Metab Care. 2002; 5: 127–132.

[3] SimopoulosAP. Evolutionary aspects of omega-3 fatty acids in the food supply. Prostaglandins Leukot Essent Fatty Acids. 1999; 60: 421–429.

[4] SimopoulosAP. The importance of the omega-6/omega-3 fatty acid ratio in cardiovascular disease and other chronic diseases. Exp Biol Med (Maywood). 2008; 233: 674–688.

[5] FuruhashiM, HotamisligilGS. Fatty acid-binding proteins: role in metabolic diseases and potential as drug targets. Nat Rev Drug Discov. 2008; 7: 489–503.

[6] PelsersMM, GlatzJF. Detection of brain injury by fatty acid-binding proteins. Clin Chem Lab Med. 2005; 43: 802–809.

[7] FigueroaJD, IllanMS, LiceroJ, CorderoK, MirandaJD, DeLM. Fatty acid binding protein 5 (FABP5) modulates docosahexaenoic acid (DHA)-induced recovery in rats undergoing spinal cord injury. J Neurotrauma. March 2016, ahead of print.

[8]   HorrocksLA, FarooquiAA. Docosahexaenoic acid in the diet: its importance in maintenance and restoration of neural membrane function. Prostaglandins Leukot Essent Fatty Acids. 2004; 70: 361–372.

[9]   GawrischK, EldhoNV, HolteLL. The structure of DHA in phospholipid membranes. Lipids. 2003; 38: 445–452.

[10] SerhanCN, KrishnamoorthyS, RecchiutiA, ChiangN. Novel anti-inflammatory—pro-resolving mediators and their receptors. Curr Top Med Chem. 2011; 11: 629–647.

[11] SerhanCN, DalliJ, ColasRA, WinklerJW, ChiangN. Protectins and maresins: new pro-resolving families of mediators in acute inflammation and resolution bioactive metabolome. Biochim Biophys Acta. 2015; 1851: 397–413.

[12] BazanNG, MolinaMF, GordonWC. Docosahexaenoic acid signalolipidomics in nutrition: significance in aging, neuroinflammation, macular degeneration, Alzheimer's, and other neurodegenerative diseases. Annu Rev Nutr. 2011; 31: 321–351.

[13] McNamaraRK, CarlsonSE. Role of omega-3 fatty acids in brain development and function: potential implications for the pathogenesis and prevention of psychopathology. Prostaglandins Leukot Essent Fatty Acids. 2006; 75: 329–349.

[14] KuratkoCN, BarrettEC, NelsonEB, SalemNJr. The relationship of docosahexaenoic acid (DHA) with learning and behavior in healthy children: a review. Nutrients. 2013; 5: 2777–2810.

[15] MartinezM, VazquezE. MRI evidence that docosahexaenoic acid ethyl ester improves myelination in generalized peroxisomal disorders. Neurology. 1998; 51: 26–32.

[16] LauritzenI, BlondeauN, HeurteauxC, WidmannC, RomeyG, LazdunskiM. Polyunsaturated fatty acids are potent neuroprotectors. EMBO J. 2000; 19: 1784–1793.

[17] DyallSC, Michael-TitusAT. Neurological benefits of omega-3 fatty acids. Neuromolecular Med. 2008; 10: 219–235.

[18] DyallSC. Long-chain omega-3 fatty acids and the brain: a review of the independent and shared effects of EPA, DPA and DHA. Front Aging Neurosci. 2015; 7: 52.

[19] RossBM, SeguinJ, SieswerdaLE. Omega-3 fatty acids as treatments for mental illness: which disorder and which fatty acid? Lipids Health Dis. 2007; 6: 21.

[20] Harris-WarrickRM. Locomotor pattern generation in the rodent spinal cord. In: JaegerD, JungR, editors. Encyclopedia of Computational Neuroscience. New York; Springer; 2013. pp. 1–15.

[21] RybakIA, DoughertyKJ, ShevtsovaNA. Organization of the mammalian locomotor CPG: review of computational model and circuit architectures based on genetically identified spinal interneurons. eNeuro. 2015; 2(5) e0069-15.2015 1–21.

[22] AzimE, JiangJ, AlstermarkB, JessellTM. Skilled reaching relies on a V2a propriospinal internal copy circuit. Nature. 2014; 508: 357–363.

[23] CroneSA, QuinlanKA, ZagoraiouL, DrohoS, RestrepoCE, LundfaldL, EndoT, SetlakJ, JessellTM, KiehnO, SharmaK. Genetic ablation of V2a ipsilateral interneurons disrupts left-right locomotor coordination in mammalian spinal cord. Neuron. 2008; 60: 70–83.

[24] ZhangY, JiSR, WuCY, FanXH, ZhouHJ, LiuGL. Observation of locomotor functional recovery in adult complete spinal rats with BWSTT using semiquantitative and qualitative methods. Spinal Cord. 2007; 45: 496–501.

[25] FernandezE, PalliniR, LaurettiL, MercantiD, SerraA, CalissanoP, PiepmeierJM, TatorCH. Spinal cord transection in adult rats — effects of local infusion of nerve growth factor on the corticospinal tract axons. Neurosurgery. 1993; 33: 889–893.

[26] BoyceVS, ParkJ, GageFH, MendellLM. Differential effects of brain-derived neurotrophic factor and neurotrophin-3 on hindlimb function in paraplegic rats. Eur J Neurosci. 2012; 35: 221–232.

[27] KubasakMD, JindrichDL, ZhongH, TakeokaA, McFarlandKC, Munoz-QuilesC, RoyRR, EdgertonVR, Ramon-CuetoA, PhelpsPE. OEG implantation and step training enhance hindlimb-stepping ability in adult spinal transected rats. Brain. 2008; 131: 264–276.

[28] RapalinoO, LazarovSpiegglerO, AgranovE, VelanGJ, YolesE, FraidakisM, SolomonA, GepsteinR, KatzA, BelkinM, HadaniM, SchwartzM. Implantation of stimulated homologous macrophages results in partial recovery of paraplegic rats. Nat Med. 1998; 4: 814–821.

[29] SlawinskaU, MajczynskiH, DjavadianR. Recovery of hindlimb motor functions after spinal cord transection is enhanced by grafts of the embryonic raphe nuclei. Exp Brain Res. 2000; 132: 27–38.

[30] FouadK, SchnellL, BungeMB, SchwabME, LiebscherT, PearseDD. Combining Schwann cell bridges and olfactory-ensheathing glia grafts with chondroitinase promotes locomotor recovery after complete transection of the spinal cord. J Neurosci. 2005; 25: 1169–1178.

[31] Lopez-ValesR, ForesJ, NavarroX, VerduE. Chronic transplantation of olfactory ensheathing cells promotes partial recovery after complete spinal cord transection in the rat. Glia. 2007; 55: 303–311.

[32] HadiB, ZhangYP, BurkeDA, ShieldsCB, MagnusonDS. Lasting paraplegia caused by loss of lumbar spinal cord interneurons in rats: no direct correlation with motor neuron loss. J Neurosurg. 2000; 93: 266–275.

[33] KingVR, HuangWL, DyallSC, CurranOE, PriestleyJV, Michael-TitusAT. Omega-3 fatty acids improve recovery, whereas omega-6 fatty acids worsen outcome, after spinal cord injury in the adult rat. J Neurosci. 2006; 26: 4672–4680.

[34] HuangWL, KingVR, CurranOE, DyallSC, WardRE, LalN, PriestleyJV, Michael-TitusAT. A combination of intravenous and dietary docosahexaenoic acid significantly improves outcome after spinal cord injury. Brain. 2007; 130: 3004–3019.

[35] LimSN, HuangW, HallJC, Michael-TitusAT, PriestleyJV. Improved outcome after spinal cord compression injury in mice treated with docosahexaenoic acid. Exp Neurol. 2013; 239: 13–27.

[36] PaternitiI, ImpellizzeriD, DiPR, EspositoE, GladmanS, YipP, PriestleyJV, Michael-TitusAT, CuzzocreaS. Docosahexaenoic acid attenuates the early inflammatory response following spinal cord injury in mice: in-vivo and in-vitro studies. J Neuroinflamm. 2014; 11: 6.

[37] BaskervilleTA, PriestleyJV, Michael-TitusAT. The effect of docosahexaenoic acid in a rat model of spinal cord injury by contusion. Soc Neurosci Abstr. 2012; 658.26/P15.

[38] HallJC, PriestleyJV, PerryVH, Michael-TitusAT. Effect of docosahexaenoic acid and eicosapentaenoic acid on the early inflammatory response following compression spinal cord injury in the rat. J Neurochem. 2012; 121: 738–750.

[39] WardRE, HuangW, CurranOE, PriestleyJV, Michael-TitusAT. Docosahexaenoic acid prevents white matter damage after spinal cord injury. J Neurotrauma. 2010; 27: 1769–1780.

[40] LiX, MurrayK, HarveyPJ, BallouEW, BennettDJ. Serotonin facilitates a persistent calcium current in motoneurons of rats with and without chronic spinal cord injury. J Neurophysiol. 2007; 97: 1236–1246.

[41] SaruhashiY, YoungW, PerkinsR. The recovery of 5-HT immunoreactivity in lumbosacral spinal cord and locomotor function after thoracic hemisection. Exp Neurol. 1996; 139: 203–213.

[42] LiuZH, YipPK, AdamsL, DaviesM, LeeJW, MichaelGJ, PriestleyJV, Michael-TitusAT. A single bolus of docosahexaenoic acid promotes neuroplastic changes in the innervation of spinal cord interneurons and motor neurons and improves functional recovery after spinal cord injury. J Neurosci. 2015; 35: 12733–12752.

[43] MontoyaCP, Campbell-HopeLJ, PembertonKD, DunnettSB. The "staircase test": a measure of independent forelimb reaching and grasping abilities in rats. J Neurosci Methods. 1991; 36: 219–228.

[44] PallierPN, PoddigheL, ZbarskyV, KostusiakM, ChoudhuryR, HartT, BurguillosMA, MusbahiO, GroenendijkM, SijbenJW, deWildeMC, QuartuM, PriestleyJV, Michael-TitusAT. A nutrient combination designed to enhance synapse formation and func-

tion improves outcome in experimental spinal cord injury. Neurobiol Dis. 2015; 82: 504–515.

[45] BareyreFM, KerschensteinerM, RaineteauO, MettenleiterTC, WeinmannO, SchwabME. The injured spinal cord spontaneously forms a new intraspinal circuit in adult rats. Nat Neurosci. 2004; 7: 269–277.

[46] PriestleyJV, Michael-TitusAT, TetzlaffW. Limiting spinal cord injury by pharmacological intervention. Handb Clin Neurol. 2012; 109: 463–484.

[47] CalderPC. Mechanisms of action of (n-3) fatty acids. J Nutr. 2012; 142: 592S–599S.

[48] UmhauJC, ZhouW, CarsonRE, RapoportSI, PolozovaA, DemarJ, HusseinN, BhattacharjeeAK, MaK, EspositoG, MajchrzakS, HerscovitchP, EckelmanWC, KurdzielKA, SalemNJr. Imaging incorporation of circulating docosahexaenoic acid into the human brain using positron emission tomography. J Lipid Res. 2009; 50: 1259–1268.

[49] Van NeervenS, MeyJ. RAR/RXR and PPAR/RXR signaling in spinal cord injury. PPAR Res. 2007; 2007: 29275.

[50] PuttaguntaR & DiGS. Retinoic acid signaling in axonal regeneration. Front Mol Neurosci. 2011; 4: 59.

[51] CurtA, van HedelHJ, KlausD, DietzV. Recovery from a spinal cord injury: significance of compensation, neural plasticity, and repair. J Neurotrauma. 2008; 25: 677–685.

[52] IchiyamaRM, CourtineG, GerasimenkoYP, YangGJ, van den BrandR, LavrovIA, ZhongH, RoyRR, EdgertonVR. Step training reinforces specific spinal locomotor circuitry in adult spinal rats. J Neurosci. 2008; 28: 7370–7375.

[53] FouadK & TetzlaffW. Rehabilitative training and plasticity following spinal cord injury. Exp Neurol. 2012; 235: 91–99.

[54] LiuG, DetloffMR, MillerKN, SantiL, HouleJD. Exercise modulates microRNAs that affect the PTEN/mTOR pathway in rats after spinal cord injury. Exp Neurol. 2012; 233: 447–456.

[55] Garcia-AliasG, FawcettJW. Training and anti-CSPG combination therapy for spinal cord injury. Exp Neurol. 2012; 235: 26–32.

[56] MaierIC, IchiyamaRM, CourtineG, SchnellL, LavrovI, EdgertonVR, SchwabME. Differential effects of anti-Nogo-A antibody treatment and treadmill training in rats with incomplete spinal cord injury. Brain. 2009; 132: 1426–1440.

3

Stem Cell Therapies for Cervical Spinal Cord Injury

Vanessa M. Doulames, Laura M. Marquardt,
Bhavaani Jayaram, Christine D. Plant and
Giles W. Plant

Abstract

Cervical-level injuries account for the majority of presented spinal cord injuries (SCIs), yet there are few therapies that successfully improve the overall quality of life for patients. Regenerative therapies aimed at ameliorating deficits in respiratory and motor function are urgently needed. Cellular transplantation strategies are a promising therapeutic avenue. These strategies seek to overcome the inhibitory environment of the injury site, increase native regenerative capacities, provide scaffolding to bridge the lesion, or replace injury-lost neurons and glia.

Numerous considerations must be taken into account, however, when designing effective cellular transplantation therapies, most notably of which is cell source. Each cell source offers its own unique attributes—both positive and negative—that directly correspond with functional outcomes and clinical translation. Here we discuss three different cell types currently used in cellular transplantation strategies to treat cervical SCIs: mesenchymal stem cells (MSCs), embryonic stem cells (ESCs), and induced pluripotent stem cells (iPSCs). By illustrating the characteristics of each cell type and outlining the studies and clinical trials in which they have been featured, we hope to provide the reader with a detailed understanding of both their capabilities and also their potential drawbacks in experimental and clinical settings.

Keywords: cervical spinal cord injury, stem cell therapies, cellular transplantation, functional outcomes, regenerative strategies

1. Introduction

1.1. The impact of cervical SCI

Spinal cord injuries (SCIs) create a formidable encumbrance on the US healthcare service with over half of all injuries occurring at the cervical level. While most causes of SCI can be attributed to accidents or violence, the incidence of cervical-specific injuries continues to rise from particularly distinctive causes [1,2]. This is in part due to the ever-increasing spectrum of injury types, such as those sustained in direct military environments or as a result of changes in tactical armor design [3–6]. Others include improvements in emergency medicine leading to better survival rates [7], the growth of the aging population as a result of advances in preventative care [8–10], and lifestyle choices leading to structural degradation of the cervical spine [11,12].

Survivors of cervical SCI are faced with dramatic life changes owing to lengthy and repeated hospitalizations and the need for full- or part-time caretakers, overall resulting in a loss of personal independence. Combined with a frequent inability to maintain employment or contribute to the workforce, patients incur substantial financial expenses—over the course of their lifetime, a 25-year-old SCI patient can expect to accrue up to $4.5 million in direct costs alone. Overall, SCI costs the nation upward of $40.5 billion annually, as per a 2009 report by the Christopher and Dana Reeve Foundation [1,2]. Although recent advances have resulted in increased survival rates, quality of life still remains poor; patients encounter a gradation of sensory deficits, respiratory deficits, motor dysfunction, and paralysis based on their specific injury location. Therapies designed to ameliorate some of these complications, even partially, are drastically needed and would make a radical impact in easing the financial, emotional, and physical burden experienced by cervical SCI patients.

1.2. The pathophysiology of cervical SCI

The cervical spinal cord contains the long tracts connecting the rostral and caudal portions of the central nervous system (CNS), as well as sensory and motor neurons. Cervical SCI in mammals initiates large zones of necrosis at the site of injury, creating gaps in the circuitry and preventing communication within the CNS. Axons within the spinal cord fail to regenerate after injury and retract toward the soma from the lesion border. Overall this culminates in crucial changes to normal upper limb function in mammals and disrupts motor function in humans resulting in paralysis and diaphragm-mediated respiration [13].

SCI is characterized by two distinct phases: primary and secondary injuries. During primary injury, the delicate spinal cord tissue is mechanically compromised due to shearing and compression forces, either by direct contact or inadvertently through manipulation of the vertebrae. This leads to mechanical injury, disruptions in vasculature and respiration, neurogenic shock, inflammation, membrane compromise, and alterations in ion and neurotransmitter levels [14–16]. While the primary injury phase leads to an immediate and often serious impairment of neurological function, it is the secondary injury phase that typically dictates the full magnitude of injury. There are approximately 25 established mechanisms to date by which this occurs, but still much ambiguity as to how these pathways converge upon each other to determine the full manifestation of injury [17,18]. Overall, this biochemical cascade activates the ischemic pathway, inflammation and immune responses, swelling, and neuronal apoptosis and leads to neurotransmitter imbalances that underlie excitotoxicity [19–25].

1.3. Regeneration and plasticity of the CNS

Prior evidence suggested that the adult mammalian CNS did not regenerate, predominantly due to the unlikely event of axonal regeneration through the inhibitory milieu of the spinal lesion [26]. However, some degree of functional recovery is often seen, possibly as a result of reorganization of spared circuitry from innate axonal sprouting of spared and intact fibers [26–28]. Experimental evidence has shown that this process can be influenced and axonal regeneration encouraged via the use of other synergistic therapies. These include the addition of neurotrophic growth factors [29–32], the deletion of inhibitory factors typically associated with the lesion [33–35], and rehabilitation regimens and physical activity [36–38]. Despite this, the innate regenerative capacities of the CNS are often overwhelmed by the extent of injury and functional recovery is limited at best.

Given SCI's multifactorial pathophysiology and the inherent complexity of the CNS, any potentially successful treatment must be effective in positively addressing multiple deficits. Cellular transplantation therapies offer an attractive means of accomplishing this by repopulating SCI-lost neurons and glia, increasing native regenerative capacities through trophic and immunomodulatory factors secreted by transplanted cells, and providing scaffolding to bridge the inhibitory milieu of the lesion site [20,29,30,32,39–43]. Furthermore, the potency of stem cells makes them an ideal candidate by circumventing the impediments of harvesting and transplanting adult neurons. By promoting neurite regeneration and replenishing appropriate cell populations, it may be possible to reconnect rostral and caudal neural circuitry and restore function.

In recent decades, the therapeutic promise of cellular intraspinal transplantation has gained significant interest and has eventuated in preliminary clinical trials. Numerous preclinical experiments have been developed to target SCI using peripheral nerve bridges, Schwann cells,

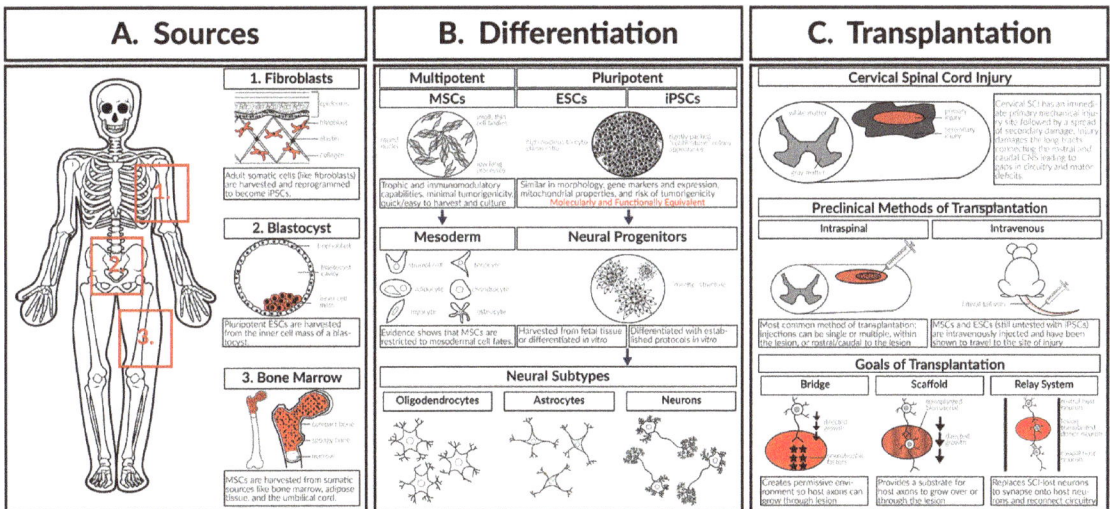

Figure 1. A summary of the different stem cell types. Panel (A) shows the origin and isolation of the cells, (B) shows their differentiation potential, and (C) describes transplantation methods used and their intended goals for treatment of cervical SCI.

olfactory glia, mesenchymal stem cells (MSCs), embryonic-derived stem cells, and induced pluripotent stem cells (iPSCs). However, the vast majority of these do not address cervical-level injury [44–52].

Here, we highlight the current literature on embryonic, mesenchymal, and induced pluripotent stem cell-based cellular transplantation with an emphasis on cervical-level SCI. We discuss the benefits and disadvantages of each cellular source, and consider possible future therapeutic avenues. **Figure 1** provides a summary of these cellular types and their origins, including transplantation methods used and their intended goals for treatment of cervical SCI.

2. Mesenchymal stem cells (MSCs)

2.1. Isolation and purification of MSCs

Transplantation of mesenchymal stem cells (MSCs), also known as bone marrow stromal cells (BMSCs) or mesenchymal progenitor cells, is a strategy currently being investigated to ameliorate the array of deleterious effects following SCI. The terms mesenchymal stromal cells and mesenchymal stem cells have been interchangeably used in the published literature; however there are demonstrable differences between the cells. Mesenchymal stem cells are a subset of stromal cells that maintain the same fibroblast morphology and specific marker expression; however they also have the potential for self-renewal and to differentiate into adipocytes, chondrocytes, and osteoblasts *in vitro* [53–55]. For cultured cells to be defined as MSCs, they should demonstrate the following: (1) adherence to plastic under culture conditions, (2) expression of CD105, CD73, and CD90, (3) lack of expression of CD45, CD34, CD14/CD11b, CD79/CD19, and HLA-DR surface markers, and (4) possession of the transdifferentiation potential to mesodermal lineages *in vitro* [56].

MSCs reside in a wide variety of tissues but are typically extracted from bone marrow and adipose tissue and to a lesser extent the umbilical cord. Their wide distribution and perivascular origin [57] account for their capability to sense and respond to injury by secreting trophic and anti-inflammatory factors [58,59]. The first report of MSCs isolation from bone marrow was by Friedenstein and colleagues. [60]. The spindle-shaped cells isolated were defined as colony-forming units (CFU) with the potential for *in vitro* culture for further transplantation *in vivo* [61]. It was only in 1999 that Pittenger and colleagues established the multi-lineage differentiation potential of MSCs into distinct mesodermal lineages [62]. Originally, Friedenstein and colleagues cultured MSCs by plastic adherence. Since then, many groups have modified this technique by expanding MSCs as a suspension culture [63–65].

Since its origin, bone marrow-derived MSC culture techniques have been continuously validated and improved. While isolation via plastic adherence is effective, the isolation of such cells does not yield a purified population of MSCs leading to varied growth kinetics and differentiation capabilities [66]. The complications of a heterogeneous population can be overcome by the purification of MSCs by using single specific surface markers such as Stro-1, CD271, Stro-3, CD73, and CD2000 [65,67]. Transplantation of MSCs, selected as above, following SCI in a rat model translated to marked improvement in functional recovery and increased tissue sparing [68].

Compared to iPSCs or embryonic stem cells (ESCs), MSCs overcome the ethical concerns of isolation, as MSCs can be extracted from one's own bone marrow or adipose tissue [69]. Recent data has indicated the principal therapeutic advantages of MSCs are their neuroprotective [70,71] and immunomodulatory [71,72] properties.

2.2. Regenerative potential of MSCs

The ubiquitous presence of MSCs around blood vessels makes them more amenable to respond to cues from tissue damage. Recent reports attribute the immunomodulatory function of MSCs as suitable for regenerative therapies and thereby tissue repair. Experimental evidence has shown that the immunomodulatory effect of MSCs is possibly due to their ability to suppress T-cell proliferation by secreting soluble factors such as TGF-beta and hepatocyte growth factor and not via apoptosis [73]. MSCs can also exert their immunomodulatory effect by shifting the balance in favor of regulatory T-cells, known suppressors of the immune system that are triggered by anti-inflammatory cytokines such as IL10. Aggarwal and Pittenger [74] co-cultured populations of immune cells with human MSCS and demonstrated that MSCs altered the secretory cytokine profile, restored balance between helper T-cells and macrophages, reduced pro-inflammatory cytokines, and increased anti-inflammatory molecules, thus favoring the induction of a tolerant anti-inflammatory phenotype [74,75]. Shifting and quenching the inflammatory response then redirects the body's resources toward tissue repair and growth [76,77]. Thus far, preclinical studies have demonstrated the potential for MSCs and their secreted factors to repair damaged tissue through their immunomodulatory and neuroprotective properties.

2.3. Treating cervical SCI with MSCs: toward clinical application

Clinically, the majority of interventions in treating SCI are pharmaceutically based and designed primarily to manage pain and control inflammation. With recent advances in stem cell therapy, there has been an increased interest in clinical studies evaluating the safety and efficacy of stem cells. MSCs are considered a favorable option for transplantation due to a number of factors: ease of isolation, rapid clinical expansion of cultures [78], ability to be cryopreserved and regenerated without loss of potency [79,80], minimal risk of tumorigenicity [81,82], multipotent capabilities, and the clinical possibility for autologous transplantation [83,84]. Furthermore, MSC transplantation has been tested widely in clinical trials and considered safe in a variety of neurological, cardiovascular, and immunological diseases [85]. As such, there is great potential for MSCs as a treatment for SCI, which has been well documented within the literature [53,68,86,87]. There are a number of clinical trials (both ongoing and completed) to test the potential of using MSCs to treat SCI (for the most current information, please refer to www.clinicaltrials.gov). Despite promising results of MSC therapies in animal SCI models and potential for clinical translation, there is yet to be an FDA approved treatment available for SCI patients.

Further investigation is needed to fully understand the basic delivery of MSCs and the mechanistic role in cervical SCI. It has not been established that engraftment and differentiation of MSCs are even needed for a therapeutic effect, and less than 1% of MSCs survive for longer than a week when systemically administered [88–90]. This survival rate would be similar in intraspinal injection. A transplantation study by Paul and colleagues compared the efficacy of hMSC engraftment when delivered either via lumbar puncture (LP), intravenous transfer (IV), or direct injection into the injury site in a rat C5 subtotal hemisection model [91]. Based on their results assessing engraftment volume (direct injection > LP > IV), glial scarring (no difference seen after 21 days of MSC transfer), and host immune response (direct injection had the highest host immune response), it can be concluded that MSC delivery via LP is a viable alternative. LP can overcome some of the difficulties of delivering MSCs in patients at the clinical setting. As a validation, a clinical trial performed by a Japanese group evaluated the effect of MSCs treatment in a single patient with a C5 fracture dislocation [92]. On day 13, he received an autologous MSC transplant via lumbar puncture and showed gradual improvement over the 6-month period in both motor and sensory scores graded according to the American Spinal Injury Association (ASIA) Scoring for International Standards for Neurological Classification of Spinal Cord Injury (ISNCSCI). Though this is a single case reported, it appears to be promising for the future of MSCs as an intervention in cervical SCI.

2.4. Sources of MSCs

2.4.1. From bone marrow stromal cells (BMSCs)

Bone marrow stem/stromal cells (BMSCs) are the most commonly used stem cell source for transplantation in experimental SCI models. These multipotent cells are derived from the heterogeneous stroma of bone marrow, which is also comprised of hematopoietic stem cells (HSC). MSCs are separated from other cells (like HSCs) by the expression of distinctive cell surface markers [53,67]. Though there has been much speculation about the transdifferentiation capacity of MSCs into neuronal and glial lineages [71,93], Hofstetter and colleagues reported that transplanted MSCs could not be induced to differentiate toward a neuronal fate, either in vitro or in vivo, in spite of the fact the MSCs displayed weak expression of NeuN (a neuronal marker) [94].

As one of the first identified sources of MSCs, BMSCs have been well studied for their anti-inflammatory, neurotrophic, and neuroprotective functions in SCI [95,96]. BMSCs transplanted into the rat spinal cord after a contusion injury demonstrated sensorimotor enhancements, partly due to their anti-inflammatory effects by attenuating activation of microglia and astrocytes [97]. To further support their therapeutic role in SCI, BMSC transplantation has been shown to reduce cavity formation, enhance axonal growth, and also prevent neuronal apoptosis [86]. While the majority of the studies have explored MSCs potential in a thoracic injury model, very few studies demonstrate their effect in a cervical SCI model; here we summarize studies relevant to cervical SCI.

One of the earliest studies to investigate transplantation within the cervical region investigated the use of rat-derived BMSCs in a combinatorial approach with cyclic adenosine monophosphate (cAMP; a neuronal stimulator) and neurotrophin-3 (NT-3; neurotrophic factor) [98]. Using a dorsal column injury as a model system, cAMP and NT-3 were injected 5 days prior to a C4 transection at L4 to precondition the DRG soma. BMSCs were then transplanted 7 days post injury. This combinatorial approach showed successful axon regeneration throughout and beyond the injury site after 12 weeks that was augmented by preconditioning with cAMP and NT-3. Despite this, functional recovery was not supported. The authors attribute the failure to the regenerating axons not reaching their target in the gracile nucleus, a major region that intercepts sensory information.

MSCs can secrete anti-inflammatory molecules and neurotrophic factors, which can lead to immunomodulation and tissue regeneration. In addition, they can also be engineered to secrete factors specific to CNS regeneration. In 2005, Lu and colleagues examined the ability of BMSCs to promote repair in the injured cord by secreting growth factors that overcome the inhibitory environment of the lesion [99]. Native or neurally induced rat-derived BMSCs were modified to either express human brain-derived neurotrophic factor (BDNF) in an acute injury or NT-3 in a chronic injury model [100]. By 1 month post transplantation within a C3 dorsal column lesion, BMSC grafts (both native and neurally induced) supported the growth of host and sensory motor axons, a finding that was augmented by either BDNF or NT-3 transduction. Transduction with neurotrophic factors substantially increased the number of coerulospinal, raphespinal, sensory, and motor axons penetrating the lesion site. Supporting these results, Novikova and colleagues transplanted BMSCs that were pretreated with Schwann-cell differentiating factors into a rat C4 hemisection model and demonstrated that BMSCs prestimulated to secrete neurotrophic factors can also contribute to inhibition of astrogliosis and the post-injury inflammatory response [101].

Another group investigated the combination of BMSCs with rat-derived neural progenitor cells (NPCs) co-transplanted in a rat C3 dorsal hemisection transection model [102]. As demyelination is a significant obstacle following SCI, the strategy was employed with the hypothesis that BMSCs would drive NPCs toward a mature oligodendrocyte lineage. In contrast with their *in vitro* data where BMSCs sufficiently redirected NPC differentiation toward an oligodendrocyte lineage, the group's *in vivo* data failed to demonstrate the same 6 weeks post transplant.

Human-derived BMSCs are a clinically attractive transplantation strategy because they can be reintroduced into patients as autografts or allografts. One preclinical study examined the transplantation of human-derived BMSCs from the iliac crest of four different healthy donors into a rat C3–C4 hemisection model [66]. Regardless of donor source, BMSCs survived and filled the lesion site with minimal migration and substantial axonal growth by 2 weeks post transplantation. By 11 weeks post transplant, no BMSCs were present within the lesion site, having been replaced by host oligodendroglial cells. Axonal infiltration into the lesion site and functional recovery varied by donor; however there was no direct correlation between the amount of axonal growth and forelimb function. One possible explanation for this is that individual donor-based distinctions in the secretory profile of BMSCs contributed to the varied outcome.

As challenging as the pitfalls within previous results may appear, there are currently two active clinical trials (Phase I NCT02574572 and Phase II/III NCT0167644) approved by the FDA to study the safety and efficacy of BMSCs transplanted in patients with chronic SCI. In conjunction with human studies, a clinical study tested the dose-dependent efficacy of autologous human-derived BMSCs in 13 patients with a mix of cervical (five patients) and thoracic (eight patients) chronic SCI. They found no deleterious effect on the patients; however only one of the 13 patients showed improvement [103]. It is possible that the absence of statistical significance can be attributed to the difference in observation of positive outcomes. For example, while one patient showed an improvement in motor power, two other patients had a patchy improvement in sensory outcome below the level of injury. At the chronic stage, the formation of glial scar tissue around the injury lesion is possibly too dense for growing axons to penetrate. While the transplantation of allogenic BMSCs was deemed safe in patients with chronic SCI, there is a need for preclinical studies to establish the mechanism of MSC's contributory role in chronic SCI.

While spinal cord injury models are in the majority represented by a contusion or hemisection injury, damage via herniated discs is also quite a common cause of disability. A herniated disc under traumatic events can lead to spinal cord injury. A discectomy is the surgical removal of the herniated nucleus pulposus of a vertebral disc to reduce pressure on the spinal cord or radiating nerves. Clinically, a discectomy is treated by fusing artificial prostheses to replace the intervertebral disc. In a preliminary proof-of-concept study utilizing an ovine model, one group sought to replicate the intervertebral disc by formulating allogeneic BMSCs with a chondrogenic agent, pentosan polysulfate, to form a cartilaginous matrix when implanted into the animal at the C3–C4 and C4–C5 levels [104]. The implant was devoid of any adverse events, and histological evidence showed predominantly cartilaginous tissue within the interbody cages. This was further confirmed by CT scans at 3 months post transplantation that showed significant bone formation in the cohort receiving BMSCs with pentosan polysulfate when compared to the cohort that received BMSCs alone. Although this particular study had its limitations, it further illustrates the potential for MSCs in preserving spinal function and advancing regenerative medicine.

2.4.2. From adipose tissue (AMSCs)

Adipose tissue is equally attractive as a cell therapy source, due to its minimally invasive harvesting procedure. From a clinical standpoint, adipose-derived stem cells (AMSCs) can easily be obtained from the large quantities of fat tissue that are removed by routine and safe procedures such as liposuction and abdominoplasties. Adipose tissue also contains supportive stroma that can be isolated and differentiated toward mesodermal lineages [105].

While a vast majority of the literature indicates that AMSCs support axonal growth, a study utilizing transplanted human-derived AMSCs in a rat C3–C4 hemisection was found to significantly reduce sprouting of the descending serotonergic fibers at the injured site [106]. The authors attributed this to several cumulative factors including enhanced survival of neurons and axons, attenuating the need for excessive sprouting, and reduced astroglial and microglial reactivity favoring the growth of the fibers into and across the transection site. Consistent with other MSC transplantation studies, there was no improvement in functional recovery despite promising microanatomical changes.

Use of AMSCs in humans has been validated for safety and toxicity in both a preclinical testing and a Phase I clinical trial [82]. It is important that every batch of stem cells prepared for transplantation into humans is processed under strict GMP conditions and the cultured cells are verified for absence of toxins and tumorigenic potential in preclinical testing. The purpose of this study was to evaluate any tumorigenic potential for hAMSCs. Twelve weeks post transplantation, the safety of transplanted AMSCs showed no significant difference in adverse events, ECG monitoring, and physical examinations. Though there was no statistical significance in ASIA score, individual patient scores showed improvement at different levels for motor and/or sensory assessment.

2.4.3. From human umbilical cord blood (UMSCs)

Human umbilical cord blood-derived MSCs (UMSCs) offer various therapeutic advantages in SCI treatment with reversal of SCI pathophysiology (downregulation of apoptotic genes and secretion of neurotrophic factors) in as little as 5 days post injury [107]. In an example using a thoracic SCI, transplantation of UMSCs was reported to have been transdifferentiated toward neuronal and oligodendroglial phenotypes. This was viewed as being a successful strategy as evidenced by improved functional motor outcome [86]. These transdifferentiated oligodendrocytes supported the injured spinal cord in remyelination by secreting neurotrophic factors [108]. UMSCs demonstrate a potential application in the treatment of SCI by their reported ability to transdifferentiate into neuronal lineages. For further information on UMSCs in thoracic injury, readers are referred to the review by Park and colleagues [109].

The first clinically based translational study to use UMSCs was in a rat model of radiation myelopathy, in which significant improvement of the microenvironment previously affected by radiation therapy was observed [110]. Radiation myelopathy is a rare, yet serious complication of cancer radiotherapy. Even though radiation myelopathy is not classified as a traditional SCI, there are many similarities in pathophysiology such as vascular damage and demyelination. This particular case study was relevant, as the group studied the efficacy of UMSCs in a radiation myelopathy model restricted to the cervical spine. Administration of the UMSCs clearly improved both microvessel and endothelial cell density, along with functional improvement in blood flow. Concurrent with other studies utilizing MSCs, UMSCs were able to reverse injury induced inflammation by reducing pro-inflammatory and increasing anti-inflammatory cytokines within the spinal cord. **Table 1** shows eight preclinical and clinical trials involving the transplantation of MSCs, describing study design, injury model, observed outcomes, and noted adverse effects.

Study and reference (PMID)	Study designs	Preclinical or clinical trials	Functional Observations	Histological/ imaging datas	Adverse events
Long-term results of spinal cord injury therapy using mesenchymal stem cells derived from bone marrow in humans (22127044)	Cells: autologous MSCs harvested from iliac bone Dosing: MSCs (8×10^6) directly injected into spinal cord and (4×10^7) were injected into intradural space Sample size: N=10 patients with ASIA class A or B injury caused by traumatic cervical SCI After 4 and 8 weeks of first injection, 5×10^7 injected via lumbar tapping Measurements: grading of motor power, MRI, electrophysiological recordings	Clinical	At 6-month follow-up: - Six out of 10 patients showed improvement in motor skills - Three out of 10 showed gradual improvement in daily activities	MRI showed a decrease in cavity size and the appearance of fiber-like low-signal intensity streaks	None observed
Intrathecal transplantation of autologous adipose-derived mesenchymal stem cells for treating spinal cord injury: a human trial (26208177)	Cells: autologous ADMSCs isolated from lipoaspirates of patient's subcutaneous fat tissue Dosing: 9×10^7 cells per patient intrathecally through lumbar tapping at day 1, 1 month, and 2 months Sample size: N=14 patients with 12 for ASIA A, 1 for B, 1 for D Six patients were injured at cervical, 1 at cervicothoracic, 6 at thoracic, and 1 at lumbar levels Measurements: MRI, hematological	Clinical	At 8-month follow-up: - ASIA motor score was improved in five patients - ASIA sensory score was improved in 10 patients - Voluntary and contraction improvement was seen in two patients - One patient showed median nerve improvement in somatosensory	MRI: no significant interval change for presence of tumorous growth EEG: no significant change after transplantation	Urinary tract infection, headache, nausea, and vomiting were observed in three patients

Study and reference (PMID)	Study designs	Preclinical or clinical trials	Functional Observations	Histological/ imaging datas	Adverse events
	parameters, electrophysiology ASIA motor/sensory scores were assessed before and after transplantation		evoked potential test		
Chronic spinal cord injury treated with transplanted autologous bone marrow-derived mesenchymal stem cells tracked by magnetic resonance imaging: a case report (25885347)	Cells: BM-derived MSCs retrieved from iliac crest were labeled with superparamagnetic iron oxide nanoparticles Dosing: intrathecal transplantation into lumbar spine with 30×10^6 cells (50:50 ratio of both labeled and unlabeled cells) After transplantation, the patient was placed in the Trendelenburg position for 24 hours Sample size: $N=1$ patient with an incomplete SCI from the atlantoaxial subluxation	Clinical	- ASIA B score did not change over 12 months - At 2 days, 6 months, and 12 months post operative, both upper and lower limbs motor score had not changes from preoperative levels - Light touch and pin prick test also did not change	MRI: showed positive signal from labeled cells in the cervical region after 48 hours No change at the structural level of injured spinal cord at any follow-up	After transplantation, patient experienced fever, headache, and myalgia with increased neurologic pain after 12 months
Transplantation of autologous bone marrow mesenchymal stem cells in the treatment of complete and chronic cervical spinal cord injury (23948102)	Cells: prepared from BM collected from iliac spine Dosing: 8×10^5 cells/μl in 25 μl slowly injected to a depth of 3 mm at multiple sites in the central dorsal area across the junction of injured and uninjured spinal cord Sample size: $N=40$ patients with complete and chronic cervical SCI divided into control and treatment groups	Clinical	- Ten patients from treatment group showed significant clinical improvement in motor, sensory, and residual urine volume - Nine patients showed changes in AIS scores - Eight out of 20 patients in the treatment group	N/A	One or two patients in the treatment group developed fever and reported headaches

Study and reference (PMID)	Study designs	Preclinical or clinical trials	Functional Observations	Histological/ imaging datas	Adverse events
			showed significant improvement in postoperative EMG		
Localized delivery of brain-derived neurotrophic factor-expressing mesenchymal stem cells enhances functional recovery following cervical spinal cord injury (25093762)	Cells: WT-MSCs or BDNF-MSCs MSCs derived from BM of adult transgenic rats expressing GFP and transduced with murine leukemia virus encoding BDNF MSCs characterized by cell surface expression of CD105 and lack of CD45 Dosing: 2 × 10⁵ cells injected intraspinally at C2 at time of injury Measurements: immunohistochemistry, electromyogram (EMG)	Preclinical: unilateral spinal cord hemisection at C2 in Sprague-Dawley rats; male	N/A	Retrograde labeling with CTB showed localization of MSCs near injection site and primarily in the white matter At day 14 after transplantation, all rats treated with BDNF-MSCs showed functional recovery of diaphragm	N/A
Bone morphogenetic proteins prevent bone marrow stromal cell-mediated oligodendroglial differentiation of transplanted adult neural progenitor cells in the injured spinal cord (23770801)	Cells: NPC isolated from sub-ventricular zone and BMSC isolated from bone marrow Dosing: immediately following the transection, cell suspensions (2 µl) containing either only BMSCs (0.6 × 10⁵ BMSCs/µl; N=5), only NPCs (1.8 × 105 NPCs/µl; N=5), or a mixture of NPCs and BMSCs (1.2 × 10⁵ NPCs/µl mixed with 0.3 × 10⁵ BMSCs/µl; N =6) were administered by a single injection into	Preclinical: C3 complete transection in adult female Fischer 344 rats	None	In vitro assays demonstrate blocking of BMP signaling enables BMSC-induced differentiation of NPCs to oligodendrocytes	

Study and reference (PMID)	Study designs	Preclinical or clinical trials	Functional Observations	Histological/ imaging datas	Adverse events
	the center of the lesion site				
Neuroprotective and growth-promoting effects of bone marrow stromal cells after cervical spinal cord injury in adult rats (21521004)	Cells: harvested from femur and tibia of rats and differentiated to a Schwann-cell phenotype Dosing: 10–12 × 10⁶ cells were injected into lateral funiculus at approx. 1 mm from the rostral and caudal site to the lesion Measurements: immunohistochemistry	Preclinical: C4 hemisection in Sprague-Dawley rats; female	N/A	At 6–8 weeks: NF-positive fibers, serotonin-positive raphespinal axons and CGRP sensory axons were seen in the injured cord	N/A
Grafting of human bone marrow stromal cells into spinal cord injury: a comparison of delivery methods (19182705)	Cells: frozen hMSC thawed and transplanted Dosing: animal groups received either 1 × 10⁶ cells transplanted via LP or IV or 1.5 × 10⁵ cells directly at injury site Measurements: histology, immunohistochemistry	Preclinical: right subtotal hemisection at C4–C5 Sprague-Dawley rats; female	N/A	Cells delivered via LP showed: - Early tissue sparing in immunostaining for GFAP - Reduced host immune response staining for ED1 (macrophage) and CD5 (pan T-cell marker)	N/A

Table 1. Tabulated summary of preclinical and clinical trials involving the transplantation of MSCs; for each trial the study design, injury model, observed outcomes and adverse effects are described.

3. Embryonic-derived stem cells (ESCs)

3.1. Derivation of embryonic stem cells

Embryonic stem cells (ESCs) represent an intriguing avenue to pursue in the race to under-stand and treat neurodegenerative pathophysiology. Their pluripotency makes them an extremely versatile option when compared to the limitations of MSCs, and the basic cell culture techniques governing them have been established for decades. ESCs are pluripotent cells derived from the inner cell mass harvested at the embryonic blastocyst stage. Unlike multipotent stem cells, such as MSCs, that are limited to mesoderm lineages, ESCs have the ability to give rise to all three germ layer lineages: the ectoderm, endoderm, and mesoderm. The capacity to generate neuronal lineages under directed conditioning makes them an ideal target for cell-based therapies of the nervous system [111–113]. Furthermore, ESCs possess the ability to self-renew, a key characteristic of stem cells that allows for a potentially indefinite source of cells.

ESCs were first harvested and cultured in the early 1980s from murine sources and eventually followed by human sources in the late 1990s [113–116]. Key differences in the *in vitro* culturing of these cells were responsible for the almost 20-year gap between the successful harvesting of murine versus human-derived ESCs. Murine ESCs are capable of surviving without the support of fibroblast feeder layers but require the addition of leukemia inhibitory factor (LIF). This led to earlier xeno-free expansion and characterization than human sources, which were later found to rely on the addition of fibroblast growth factor (FGF) to retain their pluripotency and stem cell characteristics [117].

Despite the positive attributes of ESCs, there are certain shortcomings that cannot be overlooked. Current research utilizing human-derived ESCs is still limited by the lack of chemically defined, *in vitro* culture conditions and is often dependent on the extracellular matrix and growth factor support of Matrigel substrates [118–120]. Additionally, the harvesting and culture of human-derived ESCs raise ethical concerns and extended culturing has been debated to lead to karyotypic stability. *In vivo* use of ESCs often leads to teratoma formation and the need for immunosuppressant drugs, all of which pose a problem for usage in clinical studies [111,121–123]. Current research strategies have centered around developing high-efficiency, high-purity differentiation protocols in order to generate committed or progenitor cell populations that limit their teratogenicity and enhance their therapeutic potential.

3.2. The regenerative potential of ESCs

In treating SCI, groups have looked to generate neural and glial-specific lineages such as oligodendrocytes, astrocytes, and neurons from ESCs. The majority of differentiation protocols lead to high astrocyte and oligodendrocyte populations and relatively few neurons, likely due to the proliferative capacity of the supporting glial cell types compared to neurons [40,111,124–126]. Differentiation methods developed by the McDonald and Keirstead groups have extensively researched the high-efficiency generation of oligodendrocyte progenitor cells (OPCs), which have proven useful in improving myelination and functional outcomes of increased weight support and partial hindlimb gait coordination after thoracic SCI [40,127–131].

Elegantly designed directed differentiation protocols from the Jessell research group using retinoic acid and sonic hedgehog have led to generation of spinal motor neurons from ESCs, which expressed progenitor motor neuron (pMN) marker Olig2 followed by classic motor neuron markers, Isl1, Hb9, and choline acetyltransferase (ChAT) [132]. When grafted into embryonic day 27 chick spinal cords, these cells have shown integration into the ventral spinal cord and acquire appropriate native motor pool identities [132,133], indicating a potential cell source for lost motor neuron pools after SCI. The Keirstead group has also investigated the spontaneous differentiation of human ESC-derived neural progenitor cells (NPCs) into various neuronal phenotypes such as cholinergic, serotonergic, dopaminergic (DA) and/or noradrenergic, and medium spiny striatal neurons [130,134]. Unfortunately, when ES-derived NPCs are transplanted as a heterogenic population, over-proliferation of undifferentiated stem cells can occur and potentially lead to tumor formation [135]. Further research has investigated the ways to mitigate this over-proliferation through antibiotic selection in order to generate high-purity progenitor motor neurons and committed motor neuron populations [136–138].

The first study to demonstrate that stem cells could be induced toward a cortical projection lineage utilized murine ES cells [139]. Appropriate culture conditions and *in vitro* patterning led to the generation of neural precursor cells that initially express forebrain progenitor-specific genes and later features of cortical pyramidal neurons. Most interestingly, transplantation of these cultures into various locations in the mouse brain led to area-specific axonal and dendritic growth, connectivity and integration within the host CNS, and axon extension to developmentally appropriate targets. These results suggest that it is possible to drive stem cells toward committed neural subtypes that can integrate into anatomically relevant circuits *in vivo*.

With all of these various cell populations, numerous cell-based treatment strategies for SCI have been investigated; however the overwhelming majority of these studies have been completed in thoracic injury models. Despite cervical injuries comprising more than 50% of the SCI population, very little preclinical research has been completed to date in this representative model [111].

3.3. Treating cervical SCI with ESCs

The first study to use embryonic-derived stem cells for therapy in a cervical SCI model was from Sharp and colleagues, looking at the use of human ESC-derived OPCs in a severe midline contusion cervical SCI rat model [140]. The hESC-derived OPCs used in this study were derived using the same protocol [130,131,141,142] as those used in earlier thoracic injury models from the Keirstead group [39,142] and in the Geron™-sponsored, clinical trial (first to use human ESCs as a therapeutic) that was halted in 2011 due to financial and safety concerns [143,144]. This study found that transplanting hESC-derived OPCs 7 days post injury led to a decrease in lesion area accompanied by robust white and gray matter sparing 8 weeks post transplant. Transplanted cells remained localized within the lesion epicenter with minimal rostral or caudal migration. Notably, the preservation of endogenous motor neurons was correlated with increased forelimb function. Finally, the use of transplanted hESC-derived OPCs led to differential changes in spinal cord gene expression for neurons, growth factors, apoptosis, and inflammation [140]. As such, injured animals with transplanted cells saw gene expression levels more closely matching their uninjured counterparts when compared to transplant-naïve animals. Since the discontinuation of the Geron™-sponsored thoracic injury clinical trial, Asterias Biotherapeutics, Inc., has undertaken the use of hESC AST-OPC1 cells for clinical use in a new Phase I/IIa efficacy and safety trial for cervical-level injuries (NCT02302157).

While most of the literature utilizes acute injury models to study the intervention of stem cells, one group investigated the use of hESC-derived OPCs in a rat cervical chronic injury model. In the 2013 study by Sun and colleagues, Olig2+ GFP+ OPCs derived from mouse ESCs were transplanted 4 months post rat cervical irradiation injury [145]. The irradiation injury model is a chronic injury commonly caused by radiotherapy for cancer treatment that results in the death of oligodendrocytes, which leads to severe demyelination and increased axon death. By 8 weeks post transplant, there was significantly less demyelination in addition to improved forelimb locomotor function using a clinical degree of weakness scale. Transplanted hESC-OPCs differentiated primarily into mature oligodendrocytes that expressed myelin basic protein. These cells were produced using a retinoic acid/sonic hedgehog differentiation protocol similar to the ones developed by the Jessell and Zhang groups [132,146].

The Keirstead group has also exploited the potential for ESCs to differentiate into neural lineages for use in cervical SCI treatments. They demonstrated successful use of hESC-derived progenitor motor neurons (pMNs) in a cervical SCI contusion model. The pMNs were generated using a retinoic acid differentiation protocol over 28 days and were shown to be Olig1/2+, as well as Tuj1 and Hb9 positive. Electrophysiology of these cells indicated glutamate receptors after 8 weeks in culture and could innervate both human and rodent muscle tissues. *In vivo*, reduced SCI pathology, or lesion size, and greater endogenous neuron survival and growth were observed in hESC-pMN transplanted spinal cords. Furthermore, these outcomes correlated with increased functional recovery on the balance beam task [147]. The authors did note, however, that differentiation of transplanted cells was dependent on location. Cells that were found in the distal ventral horn led to increased differentiation, whereas cells confined to the site of injury reverted to a progenitor state.

Other embryonic or fetal-derived tissues have been used in spinal cord injury therapies, including whole fetal spinal cord transplants (pioneered by Reier and Anderson) and fetal neural progenitor/stem cells taken from brain and spinal tissue [51,111,123,148–157]. In the study by Diener and Bregman, transplantation of fetal spinal cord tissues into cervical hemisections led to supraspinal growth, axon projections, improved skilled forelimb function indicating transplanted cell survival, and potential local circuit formation. Further investigation of fetal spinal cord lineage-restricted NPCs by various groups has indicated differentiation of transplanted cells into all three neural lineages, in both cervical and thoracic level injuries, with long distance cell migration and axon growth leading to functional improvement [123,148–151,158]. Two clinical trials have begun since 2013 investigating the use of fetal-derived tissues for spinal cord injury [144]. StemCells, Inc.® have begun a safety and efficacy study using human-derived CNS-stem cells (proprietary source) in cervical SCI after completing a thoracic injury trial [159]. Neuralstem, Inc., is also investigating the use of fetal stem cells in SCI [160,161] after promising results using such cells in ALS treatment. This trial, however, is determining the efficacy of these cells in a thoracic injury model. While these cells have proven useful in improving functional outcomes after SCI in preclinical trials, they are subject to the same ethical concerns as those for ESCs and have limited differentiation capacity in comparison [162].

In treating SCI, ESCs demonstrate great potential in promoting axon regeneration and functional recovery, but the lack of full characterization of cell safety, efficacy, and phenotype has significantly limited their clinical applications. Furthermore, the use of ESCs in cervical SCI models is limited to less than a handful of peer-reviewed studies. As cervical injuries are becoming more prevalent, future studies must be designed that better replicate clinical injuries in order to more accurately test cell therapeutic strategies.

4. Induced pluripotent stem cells (iPSCs)

4.1. Derivation of iPSCs

Induced pluripotent stem cells (iPSCs) are created by reprogramming adult somatic fibroblasts to revert to a pluripotent stem cell state initially via retroviral delivery of Oct3/4, Sox2, c-Myc, and Klf4 [163–165]. Now iPSCs can be generated via multiple processes, each with its own merits and limitations. Viral transduction is easy to use and reproducible, yields iPSCs efficiently, and is controlled. However there is an increased risk of insertional mutagenesis and transgene reactivation, incomplete splicing, and clone-to-clone variation [166–168]. Reprogramming factors can also be fused to cell-penetrating peptides or introduced through plasmids, which requires no genomic modification but is also a time consuming and potentially inefficient process [169]. Finally iPSCs can be induced via mRNA introduction, which is a highly effective and rapid method; it also requires no genomic modification and is deemed safe due to the transient nature of mRNA. However, repeated transfections are typically required [170,171].

While MSCs are hindered by their limited potency and the harvesting of ESCs is subject to ethical constraints, the pluripotency and source of iPSCs circumvent some of these issues, therefore making them a promising alternative in cellular transplantation therapies. iPSCs share many similarities with ESCs and provide a comparative alternative in that they have the same morphology, gene markers, and potential to form teratomas (ability to differentiate into all three germ layers) [163,165]. Furthermore, the use of iPSCs opens up new possibilities for clinical consideration—ethical concerns are diminished and, in the case of potential transplants, cells can be harvested directly from the patient, therefore avoiding the need for immunosuppression.

4.2. Cell reprogramming technologies for controlled differentiation

There has been a strong motivation to create iPSC differentiation protocols that drive stem cells toward the three main neural lineages *in vitro*. Methods to generate functional neurons have been of particular interest so as to study the differences in neuronal networks in both healthy and impaired states [172–177]. In one report, mature human fibroblasts were directly programmed into synaptically active functional neurons via a cocktail of miR-124, BRN2, and MYT1L [178]. An additional group found that Ascl1 (which has pioneer factor properties) in conjunction with BRN2, and MYT1L, successfully drove murine fibroblasts into neuronal cells with appropriate morphology, expression, and formation of functional synapses [179]. One report demonstrated that the overexpression of neurogenin 2 efficiently transformed iPSCs into functional neurons that were able to spontaneously form excitatory synaptic networks. Furthermore, these networks both synaptically integrate once transplanted into the mouse brain and exhibit plasticity [180]. The majority of research utilizes iPSCs driven toward a neural progenitor state [181,182]; however iPSC differentiation has also been useful in disease modeling. As an example, midbrain dopaminergic (DA) neuron phenotypes have been generated, which has been particularly useful in studying Parkinson's disease (PD), typically characterized by the loss of these DA neurons [183–186]. In one study by the Pera group, a stable iPSC line was derived from a PD patient that carried the most common PD-associated genetic mutation and differentiated into midbrain DA neurons. These iPSC-derived DA neurons exhibited classic hallmarks of PD-related damage including accumulation of α-synuclein and oxidative stress, susceptibility to H_2O_2-induced CASP3 activation, and sensitivity to 6-OHDA and proteasome inhibition. Additionally, other groups have shown that iPSCs can be successfully driven toward glutamatergic, GABAergic, motor, and retinal neuron phenotypes [187–199]. While not specific to SCI, these results demonstrate that developing differentiation protocols capable of generating specific neural subtypes can open up new research avenues in understanding and creating therapies for neuropathologies.

There is also interest in reliably driving iPSCs toward functional glial subtypes, as glial cells are heavily affected in the process of neurodegeneration. In a study by Krencik and Zhang, exogenous patterning molecules were used to transform iPSCs into a neuroepithelial phenotype. From there, administration of mitogens allowed for the generation of astroglial progenitors, which could then be further differentiated into functional astrocytes via ciliary neurotrophic factor [200]. Another protocol utilized the forced expression of Sox10, Olig2, and Zfb536 to directly reprogram rodent fibroblasts into oligodendrocyte precursor cells. The resulting population of precursors exhibited typical morphology and gene expression and gave rise to mature oligodendrocytes that could ensheath dorsal root ganglion cells *in vitro* and form myelin *in vivo* [201].

The intended goal behind SCI therapies is to ameliorate damage and restore the circuitry within the CNS. Cellular transplantation offers an innovative means in accomplishing this, but is obviously extremely dependent upon the characteristics and capabilities of the transplanted cell type. Driving human iPSCs toward neuronal lineages via reproducible and robust differentiation protocols represents a practical interface between developmental neurobiology and SCI research; it may be possible to tailor iPSCs toward a more developmentally appropriate, specific neuronal cell type capable of restoring CNS connectivity rather than the uncharacterized progenitor populations previously used with limited functional recovery.

4.3. Treating cervical SCI with iPSCs

Similar to MSC and ESC-focused SCI therapies, there is a scarcity of targeted preclinical therapies for SCI using iPSC transplantation. Therapies do show positive outcomes yet they are limited in number; to date there are only five published studies using either rodent or simian models of thoracic SCI [202]. In these studies, iPSCs were driven toward neural stem spheres [203], neural stem cells (NSCs) [202,204], and neurospheres [205,206] with all except one study experiencing amelioration of the inhibitory nature of the lesion site, synaptic integration of transplanted cells, and significant functional improvement in transplanted animals.

Therapies targeting cervical SCI are equally as limited. There are four published studies to date that have examined acute, subacute, and chronic iPSC transplantation following cervical SCI. Li and colleagues evaluated respiratory function following transplantation of iPSC-derived astrocytes engineered to overexpress GLT1, an astroglial glutamate transporter [207]. Both rats and mice underwent a C4 contusion injury resulting in chronic diaphragm dysfunction and phrenic motor neuron deterioration. Immediately post injury, subjects received two separate intraspinal injections rostral and caudal to the lesion within the ventral horn. At time points ranging from 2 days to 4 weeks post transplant, it was demonstrated that transplanted grafts survived and differentiated into GFAP-positive astrocytes, were not tumorigenic, and had less than 10% proliferation (evidenced by Ki67 staining). Furthermore, lesion area and volume were reduced within 1 mm rostral and caudal to the lesion epicenter and innervation of the diaphragm neuromuscular junction was preserved in animals that had received iPSC-derived astrocyte transplants that overexpressed GLT1. Through analysis of spontaneous electromyogram (EMG) activity, GLT1-overexpressing astrocyte transplants significantly magnified EMG amplitude in the dorsal region of the hemidiaphragm, further demonstrating preservation of diaphragmatic respiratory function.

Another study by Lu and colleagues examined the effect of human iPSC-derived NSCs harvested from an elderly donor in a C5 lateral hemisection rat model [208]. While the chosen cell population was minimally characterized, *in vitro* analysis demonstrated reduced expression of Tra1-81 and SSEA4 (pluripotency markers) and maintained expression of nestin and Sox2 (NSC-associated markers). Two weeks post injury, NSCs were intraspinally co-transplanted with a fibrin matrix and a raft of growth factors. By 3 months post transplantation, there was evidence that the grafted cells had survived, distributed throughout the lesion, and integrated with host axons. The majority of grafted cells expressed NeuN and mature neuronal markers MAP2 and Tuj1 alongside mature astrocytic marker GFAP, suggesting preferential differentiation into neuronal and astrocytic lineages. There was also evidence of proliferation and spinal motor neuron identity within a small percentage of transplanted cells via the expression of Ki67 and ChAT, respectively. Most notably, a remarkable amount of axonal growth was present extending from the lesion site toward the olfactory bulbs and lumbar spine sections. Despite robust axonal growth, no behavioral recovery was observed.

In consideration of the substantial lack of existing chronic cervical SCI data, Nutt and colleagues investigated an early chronic injury model mimicking the deficits seen in human injury [209]. Four weeks following a cervical contusion injury at C4, iPSC-derived neural progenitor cells and fibroblasts were co-transplanted rostral and caudal to the lesion in a rat model. Immunohistochemical analysis suggested the differentiation of transplanted cells into mature neurons as well as the intermingling of the host CNS with transplanted cells, as evidenced by NeuN/FOX-3 labeling. Despite interactions between host and donor cells, transplanted cells did not express glutamate receptors. Furthermore, transplanted cells were not positive for serotonin but did express GABA and were shown co-localized with host positive choline acetyltransferase. Behavioral recovery was weak; grasping and weight bearing were only slightly improved by transplants.

	MSCs	ESCs	iPSCs
Source	Bone marrow, adipose, umbilical cord	Fetal tissue	Somatic (adult) cells
Lineage differentiation	Mesodermal lineage	All three germ layers— endoderm, mesoderm, and ectoderm	All three germ layers— endoderm, mesoderm, and ectoderm
Derivation	Purified by surface markers from adult tissue	Embryonic (inner cell mass of blastocyst)	Induced or reprogrammed to "stemness"
Ease of isolation	Easily accessible sources	Difficult; isolated from fetal tissue	Easily accessible sources (e.g., skin)
Differentiation potential	Multipotent	Pluripotent	Pluripotent
Ethical issues	Minimal; cells can be isolated from the patient	Strong concerns	Minimal; even skin cells can be induced to be pluripotent
Axonal regrowth	Yes; by tissue sparing and neuroprotection	Yes; by transdifferentiation	Yes; by transdifferentiation
Functional outcome	Mild to moderate	Moderate	Mild to moderate
Immunomodulatory	Yes	Low	Low
Immunogenicity/ autologous	Low; safe for autologous transplantation	High; often requires immunosuppression	Low; safe for autologous transplantation
Tumorigenicity	No tumor formation	Teratoma formation	Teratoma formation
Clinical trial	Advanced to Phase III	Advanced to Phase II	Preclinical only

Table 2. A comparative scheme of the characteristics of MSCs, ESCs and iPSCs described in this chapter.

In contrast, Kobayashi and colleagues examined the safety and efficacy of iPSC-derived NSC transplants in a simian model of cervical SCI [210]. Human iPSCs were cultured and induced to form neurospheres and passaged a secondary and tertiary time prior to transplantation. Adult female marmosets were given a moderate contusion at the C5 level and received an intraspinal injection of cultured iPSC-neurospheres 9 days post injury at the lesion site. By 12 weeks post transplant, hematoxylin-eosin staining revealed that the grafted cells survived and were positive for NeuN, GFAP, and Olig 1 indicating differentiation into all three neural subtypes. Additionally, animals that received transplants had reduced cystic cavity size, no evidence of tumorigenicity, increased angiogenesis, and a higher amount of neurofilaments and descending motor axons at the lesion center. Severe demyelination was evident surrounding the lesion site in both transplanted and control groups; however, the amount was significantly exacerbated in animals that did not receive cellular transplantation. These findings were further supported by MRI and myelin mapping in which myelin sparing was more evident in the transplanted group and an intramedullary high-signal intensity area in the lesion site of the control group. Calcitonin-generated peptide fibers, which are involved in spinal pain mechanisms, did not differ between transplanted and control groups. In nonhuman primates, contusion at the C5 level in a severed central cord injury model leads to tetraplegia with an expected gradual improvement in motor function. By 8 weeks post injury, there were significant differences in the open field test, bar grip strength test, and cage climbing tests between transplanted and control groups, which stayed consistent throughout the study indicating some level of functional recovery due to transplantation. Promising results from the various cell-based therapies have demonstrated varying degrees of axonal regeneration and functional recovery. **Table 2** provides a summary of the characteristics of MSC, ESC, and iPSC types and also notes their functional outcomes, tumorigenicity, and clinical trial stage to date.

5. Summary and conclusions

Great care and consideration must be taken when choosing an optimal stem cell type as a potential cellular transplantation treatment for cervical SCIs. Of the three main stem cell types discussed here, there are distinct advantages and disadvantages to each. The use of MSCs in treating nervous system injuries remains a hotly debated topic due to their limited survival, differentiation potential, and functional recovery outcomes. Nevertheless, their immunomodulatory properties and growth factor secretion make them potentially beneficial for use in combinatorial strategies especially if delivered noninvasively. ESCs offer significantly more differentiation potential for neural applications than adult stem cells and have the added benefit of promoting functional recovery in cervical SCI models. However, the lack of detailed cell characterization, need for immunosuppression, and overall ethical concerns have led to only a single cervical SCI clinical trial. Moreover, the use of ESCs in preclinical cervical SCI studies is limited to only two ESC-derived phenotypes (OPCs and pMNs). Significant research must still be performed to fully explore alternative appropriate cell types that can potentially promote functional regeneration. Finally iPSCs, the newest technology in stem cell sources, propose an interesting alternative to fate-limited MSCs and ethically restricted ESCs in treating cervical SCI. Promising preclinical data has indicated iPSC-based therapies can improve functional outcomes after injury; however, their recent discovery highlights the need for careful characterization and exploration of secure differentiation protocols. Further studies must still be completed before iPSCs can be approved for clinical applications.

While stem cell transplantation therapies have shown promise in promoting post-injury regeneration, both anatomical and functional recovery still remain imperfect; no preclinical or clinical study to date has dramatically restored significant recovery in patients. Experimental evidence has shown that native regeneration and plasticity occur in limited amounts following injury. These innate processes can be enhanced via the addition of neurotrophic and immunomodulatory factors, the removal of lesion-associated inhibitory factors, and injury-appropriate rehabilitation regimens and physical activity. It would be of great interest to determine whether combinatorial approaches utilizing stem cell transplantation in conjunction with the strategies described above provides a synergistic effect within the living system. Furthermore, the vast majority of cell transplantation studies utilize cell populations driven toward immature final phenotypes. The pluripotent capabilities of ESCs and iPSCs provide the freedom to drive these cell types toward numerous definitive lineages or ages. This, however, will be defined by developing appropriate differentiation protocols that can be used in both preclinical and clinical settings. It is possible that transplanting more mature cells results in the establishment and integration of meaningful circuitry within the host nervous system to restore and promote functional recovery.

The broad scope of stem cell therapies offers a myriad of therapeutic potential. However, due to the limited number of preclinical and clinical studies, extensive logistical questions remain regarding how to optimize their usage. Nonetheless, the great strides made in designing and improving effective stem cell therapies for enhancing function promises an exciting future for the field of spinal cord injury repair.

Author details

Vanessa M. Doulames, Laura M. Marquardt, Bhavaani Jayaram, Christine D. Plant and Giles W. Plant*

*Address all correspondence to: gplant@stanford.edu

Department of Neurosurgery, Stanford University School of Medicine, Stanford, CA, USA

References

[1] Cahill, A., et al. *One Degree of Separation: Paralysis and Spinal Cord Injury in the United States*, 2009, Christopher and Dana Reeves Paralysis Resource Center, p. 1–28.

[2] National Spinal Cord Injury Statistical Center. *Facts and Figures at a Glance*, 2015, University of Alabama at Birmingham: Birmingham, AL.

[3] Wagner, C.S. and A.R. Lehman, *Cervical spine and neck injuries*, in *Musculoskeletal Injuries in the Military*, L.K. Cameron and D.B. Owens, Editors, 2016, Springer New York: New York, NY, p. 229–45.

[4] Breeze, J., et al., *Defining combat helmet coverage for protection against explosively propelled fragments*. J R Army Med Corps, 2015. 161(1): p. 9–13.

[5] Inoue, T., et al., *Combined SCI and TBI: recovery of forelimb function after unilateral cervical spinal cord injury (SCI) is retarded by contralateral traumatic brain injury (TBI), and ipsilateral TBI balances the effects of SCI on paw placement.* Exp Neurol, 2013. 248: p. 136–47.

[6] Yoganandan, N., et al., *Cervical spine injury biomechanics: applications for under body blast loadings in military environments.* Clin Biomech (Bristol, Avon), 2013. 28(6): p. 602–9.

[7] Ropper, A.E., M.T. Neal, and N. Theodore, *Acute management of traumatic cervical spinal cord injury.* Pract Neurol, 2015. 15(4): p. 266–72.

[8] Laing, A.C., et al., *The effects of age on the morphometry of the cervical spinal cord and spinal column in adult rats: an MRI-based study.* Anat Rec (Hoboken), 2014. 297(10): p. 1885–95.

[9] Tetreault, L., et al., *Degenerative cervical myelopathy: a spectrum of related disorders affecting the aging spine.* Neurosurgery, 2015. 77(Suppl 4): p. S51–67.

[10] Wang, T.Y., et al., *Risk assessment and characterization of 30-day perioperative myocardial infarction following spine surgery: a retrospective analysis of 1346 consecutive adult patients.* Spine (Phila Pa 1976), 2016. 41(5): p. 438–44.

[11] Satyanand, V., et al., *Effects of yogasanas on cervical spondylosis.* IAIM, 2015. 2(7): p. 6–10.

[12] Smith, H.E., et al., *Spine care: evaluation of the efficacy and cost of emerging technology.* Am J Med Qual, 2009. 24(6 Suppl): p. 25S–31S.

[13] Gensel, J.C., et al., *Behavioral and histological characterization of unilateral cervical spinal cord contusion injury in rats.* J Neurotrauma, 2006. 23(1): p. 36–54.

[14] Peitzman, A.B., *The trauma manual: trauma and acute care surgery.* 4th ed, C.W.S.M. Rhodes, D.M. Yealy, T.C. Fabian, and A.B. Peitzman, Editors, 2012, Lippincott Williams & Wilkins. Philidelphia. 4th Ed. 2012. pgs:1–824

[15] Sabapathy, V., G. Tharion, and S. Kumar, *Cell therapy augments functional recovery subsequent to spinal cord injury under experimental conditions.* Stem Cells Int, 2015. 2015: p. 132172.

[16] Newman, M.F., L.A. Fleisher, and M.P. Fink, *Perioperative Medicine: Managing for Outcome,* 2008, Elsevier Health Sciences. United States. 2007. pgs:1–752

[17] Ramer, L.M., M.S. Ramer, and J.D. Steeves, *Setting the stage for functional repair of spinal cord injuries: a cast of thousands.* Spinal Cord, 2005. 43(3): p. 134–61.

[18] Tator, C.H., *Biology of neurological recovery and functional restoration after spinal cord injury.* Neurosurgery, 1998. 42(4): p. 696–707; discussion 707-8.

[19] Beattie, M.S., A.A. Farooqui, and J.C. Bresnahan, *Review of current evidence for apoptosis after spinal cord injury.* J Neurotrauma, 2000. 17(10): p. 915–25.

[20] Donnelly, D.J. and P.G. Popovich, *Inflammation and its role in neuroprotection, axonal regeneration and functional recovery after spinal cord injury.* Exp Neurol, 2008. 209(2): p. 378–88.

[21] Dumont, R.J., et al., *Acute spinal cord injury, part I: pathophysiologic mechanisms.* Clin Neuropharmacol, 2001. 24(5): p. 254–64.

[22] Hausmann, O.N., *Post-traumatic inflammation following spinal cord injury.* Spinal Cord, 2003. 41(7): p. 369–78.

[23] Lu, J., K.W. Ashwell, and P. Waite, *Advances in secondary spinal cord injury: role of apoptosis.* Spine (Phila Pa 1976), 2000. 25(14): p. 1859–66.

[24] Mautes, A.E., et al., *Vascular events after spinal cord injury: contribution to secondary pathogenesis.* Phys Ther, 2000. 80(7): p. 673–87.

[25] Park, E., A.A. Velumian, and M.G. Fehlings, *The role of excitotoxicity in secondary mechanisms of spinal cord injury: a review with an emphasis on the implications for white matter degeneration.* J Neurotrauma, 2004. 21(6): p. 754–74.

[26] Horner, P.J. and F.H. Gage, *Regenerating the damaged central nervous system.* Nature, 2000. 407(6807): p. 963–70.

[27] Bernstein, J.J. and M.E. Bernstein, *Axonal regeneration and formation of synapses proximal to the site of lesion following hemisection of the rat spinal cord.* Exp Neurol, 1971. 30(2): p. 336–51.

[28] Ramer, M.S., J.V. Priestley, and S.B. McMahon, *Functional regeneration of sensory axons into the adult spinal cord.* Nature, 2000. 403(6767): p. 312–6.

[29] Bregman, B.S., et al., *Neurotrophic factors increase axonal growth after spinal cord injury and transplantation in the adult rat.* Exp Neurol, 1997. 148(2): p. 475–94.

[30] Grill, R., et al., *Cellular delivery of neurotrophin-3 promotes corticospinal axonal growth and partial functional recovery after spinal cord injury.* J Neurosci, 1997. 17(14): p. 5560–72.

[31] McTigue, D.M., et al., *Neurotrophin-3 and brain-derived neurotrophic factor induce oligodendrocyte proliferation and myelination of regenerating axons in the contused adult rat spinal cord.* J Neurosci, 1998. 18(14): p. 5354–65.

[32] Ye, J.H. and J.D. Houle, *Treatment of the chronically injured spinal cord with neurotrophic factors can promote axonal regeneration from supraspinal neurons.* Exp Neurol, 1997. 143(1): p. 70–81.

[33] Kim, G.M., et al., *Tumor necrosis factor receptor deletion reduces nuclear factor-kappaB activation, cellular inhibitor of apoptosis protein 2 expression, and functional recovery after traumatic spinal cord injury.* J Neurosci, 2001. 21(17): p. 6617–25.

[34] Nishio, Y., et al., *Deletion of macrophage migration inhibitory factor attenuates neuronal death and promotes functional recovery after compression-induced spinal cord injury in mice.* Acta Neuropathol, 2009. 117(3): p. 321–8.

[35] Simonen, M., et al., *Systemic deletion of the myelin-associated outgrowth inhibitor Nogo-A improves regenerative and plastic responses after spinal cord injury.* Neuron, 2003. 38(2): p. 201–11.

[36] Engesser-Cesar, C., et al., *Voluntary wheel running improves recovery from a moderate spinal cord injury.* J Neurotrauma, 2005. 22(1): p. 157–71.

[37] Hamid, S. and R. Hayek, *Role of electrical stimulation for rehabilitation and regeneration after spinal cord injury: an overview.* Eur Spine J, 2008. 17(9): p. 1256–69.

[38] Smith, R.R., et al., *Effects of swimming on functional recovery after incomplete spinal cord injury in rats.* J Neurotrauma, 2006. 23(6): p. 908–19.

[39] Keirstead, H.S., et al., *Human embryonic stem cell-derived oligodendrocyte progenitor cell transplants remyelinate and restore locomotion after spinal cord injury.* J Neurosci, 2005. 25(19): p. 4694–705.

[40] McDonald, J.W., et al., *Transplanted embryonic stem cells survive, differentiate and promote recovery in injured rat spinal cord.* Nat Med, 1999. 5(12): p. 1410–2.

[41] Popovich, P.G., et al., *Depletion of hematogenous macrophages promotes partial hindlimb recovery and neuroanatomical repair after experimental spinal cord injury.* Exp Neurol, 1999. 158(2): p. 351–65.

[42] Thuret, S., L.D. Moon, and F.H. Gage, *Therapeutic interventions after spinal cord injury.* Nat Rev Neurosci, 2006. 7(8): p. 628–43.

[43] Chopp, M., et al., *Spinal cord injury in rat: treatment with bone marrow stromal cell transplantation.* Neuroreport, 2000. 11(13): p. 3001–5.

[44] Barry, F.P. and J.M. Murphy, *Mesenchymal stem cells: clinical applications and biological characterization.* Int J Biochem Cell Biol, 2004. 36(4): p. 568–84.

[45] Carpenter, M.K., E. Rosler, and M.S. Rao, *Characterization and differentiation of human embryonic stem cells.* Cloning Stem Cells, 2003. 5(1): p. 79–88.

[46] Cummings, B.J., et al., *Human neural stem cells differentiate and promote locomotor recovery in spinal cord-injured mice.* Proc Natl Acad Sci U S A, 2005. 102(39): p. 14069–74.

[47] Plant, G.W., M.L. Bates, and M.B. Bunge, *Inhibitory proteoglycan immunoreactivity is higher at the caudal than the rostral Schwann cell graft-transected spinal cord interface.* Mol Cell Neurosci, 2001. 17(3): p. 471–87.

[48] Ramer, L.M., et al., *Peripheral olfactory ensheathing cells reduce scar and cavity formation and promote regeneration after spinal cord injury.* J Comp Neurol, 2004. 473(1): p. 1–15.

[49] Ruitenberg, M.J., et al., *Viral vector-mediated gene expression in olfactory ensheathing glia implants in the lesioned rat spinal cord.* Gene Ther, 2002. 9(2): p. 135–46.

[50] Snyder, E.Y. and Y.D. Teng, *Stem cells and spinal cord repair.* N Engl J Med, 2012. 366(20): p. 1940–2.

[51] Reier, P.J., B.S. Bregman, and J.R. Wujek, *Intraspinal transplantation of embryonic spinal cord tissue in neonatal and adult rats.* J Comp Neurol, 1986. 247(3): p. 275–96.

[52] Reubinoff, B.E., et al., *Neural progenitors from human embryonic stem cells.* Nat Biotechnol, 2001. 19(12): p. 1134–40.

[53] Hodgetts, S.I., P.J. Simmons, and G.W. Plant, *Human mesenchymal precursor cells (Stro-1(+)) from spinal cord injury patients improve functional recovery and tissue sparing in an acute spinal cord injury rat model.* Cell Transplant, 2013. 22(3): p. 393–412.

[54] Horwitz, E.M., et al., *Clarification of the nomenclature for MSC: The International Society for Cellular Therapy position statement.* Cytotherapy, 2005. 7(5): p. 393–5.

[55] Bianco, P., et al., *The meaning, the sense and the significance: translating the science of mesenchymal stem cells into medicine.* Nat Med, 2013. 19(1): p. 35–42.

[56] Dominici, M., et al., *Minimal criteria for defining multipotent mesenchymal stromal cells. The International Society for Cellular Therapy position statement.* Cytotherapy, 2006. 8(4): p. 315–7.

[57] Crisan, M., et al., *A perivascular origin for mesenchymal stem cells in multiple human organs.* Cell Stem Cell, 2008. 3(3): p. 301–13.

[58] Bai, L., et al., *Hepatocyte growth factor mediates mesenchymal stem cell-induced recovery in multiple sclerosis models.* Nat Neurosci, 2012. 15(6): p. 862–70.

[59] Honczarenko, M., et al., *Human bone marrow stromal cells express a distinct set of biologically functional chemokine receptors.* Stem Cells, 2006. 24(4): p. 1030–41.

[60] Friedenstein, A.J., R.K. Chailakhjan, and K.S. Lalykina, *The development of fibroblast colonies in monolayer cultures of guinea-pig bone marrow and spleen cells.* Cell Tissue Kinet, 1970. 3(4): p. 393–403.

[61] Friedenstein, A.J., et al., *Stromal cells responsible for transferring the microenvironment of the hemopoietic tissues. Cloning in vitro and retransplantation in vivo.* Transplantation, 1974. 17(4): p. 331–40.

[62] Pittenger, M.F., et al., *Multilineage potential of adult human mesenchymal stem cells.* Science, 1999. 284(5411): p. 143–7.

[63] Castro-Malaspina, H., et al., *Characterization of human bone marrow fibroblast colony-forming cells (CFU-F) and their progeny.* Blood, 1980. 56(2): p. 289–301.

[64] Goshima, J., V.M. Goldberg, and A.I. Caplan, *The osteogenic potential of culture-expanded rat marrow mesenchymal cells assayed in vivo in calcium phosphate ceramic blocks.* Clin Orthop Relat Res, 1991(262): p. 298–311.

[65] Simmons, P.J. and B. Torok-Storb, *Identification of stromal cell precursors in human bone marrow by a novel monoclonal antibody, STRO-1.* Blood, 1991. 78(1): p. 55–62.

[66] Neuhuber, B., et al., *Axon growth and recovery of function supported by human bone marrow stromal cells in the injured spinal cord exhibit donor variations.* Brain Res, 2005. 1035(1): p. 73–85.

[67] Kfoury, Y. and D.T. Scadden, *Mesenchymal cell contributions to the stem cell niche.* Cell Stem Cell, 2015. 16(3): p. 239–53.

[68] Hodgetts, S.I., P.J. Simmons, and G.W. Plant, *A comparison of the behavioral and anatomical outcomes in sub-acute and chronic spinal cord injury models following treatment with human mesenchymal precursor cell transplantation and recombinant decorin.* Exp Neurol, 2013. 248: p. 343–59.

[69] Gronthos, S., et al., *Surface protein characterization of human adipose tissue-derived stromal cells.* J Cell Physiol, 2001. 189(1): p. 54–63.

[70] Torres-Espin, A., et al., *Neuroprotection and axonal regeneration after lumbar ventral root avulsion by re-implantation and mesenchymal stem cells transplant combined therapy.* Neurotherapeutics, 2013. 10(2): p. 354–68.

[71] Uccelli, A., L. Moretta, and V. Pistoia, *Mesenchymal stem cells in health and disease.* Nat Rev Immunol, 2008. 8(9): p. 726–36.

[72] Bai, L., et al., *Human bone marrow-derived mesenchymal stem cells induce Th2-polarized immune response and promote endogenous repair in animal models of multiple sclerosis.* Glia, 2009. 57(11): p. 1192–203.

[73] Di Nicola, M., et al., *Human bone marrow stromal cells suppress T-lymphocyte proliferation induced by cellular or nonspecific mitogenic stimuli.* Blood, 2002. 99(10): p. 3838–43.

[74] Aggarwal, S. and M.F. Pittenger, *Human mesenchymal stem cells modulate allogeneic immune cell responses.* Blood, 2005. 105(4): p. 1815–22.

[75] Kong, Q.F., et al., *Administration of bone marrow stromal cells ameliorates experimental autoimmune myasthenia gravis by altering the balance of Th1/Th2/Th17/Treg cell subsets through the secretion of TGF-beta.* J Neuroimmunol, 2009. 207(1-2): p. 83–91.

[76] Tidball, J.G. and S.A. Villalta, *Regulatory interactions between muscle and the immune system during muscle regeneration.* Am J Physiol Regul Integr Comp Physiol, 2010. 298(5): p. R1173–87.

[77] Tollervey, J.R. and V.V. Lunyak, *Adult stem cells: simply a tool for regenerative medicine or an additional piece in the puzzle of human aging?* Cell Cycle, 2011. 10(24): p. 4173–6.

[78] Sekiya, I., et al., *Expansion of human adult stem cells from bone marrow stroma: conditions that maximize the yields of early progenitors and evaluate their quality.* Stem Cells, 2002. 20(6): p. 530–41.

[79] Kotobuki, N., et al., *Cultured autologous human cells for hard tissue regeneration: preparation and characterization of mesenchymal stem cells from bone marrow.* Artif Organs, 2004. 28(1): p. 33–9.

[80] Lee, M.W., et al., *Isolation of mesenchymal stem cells from cryopreserved human umbilical cord blood.* Int J Hematol, 2005. 81(2): p. 126–30.

[81] Lalu, M.M., et al., *Safety of cell therapy with mesenchymal stromal cells (SafeCell): a systematic review and meta-analysis of clinical trials.* PLoS One, 2012. 7(10): p. e47559.

[82] Ra, J.C., et al., *Safety of intravenous infusion of human adipose tissue-derived mesenchymal stem cells in animals and humans.* Stem Cells Dev, 2011. 20(8): p. 1297–308.

[83] Fouillard, L., et al., *Infusion of allogeneic-related HLA mismatched mesenchymal stem cells for the treatment of incomplete engraftment following autologous haematopoietic stem cell transplantation.* Leukemia, 2007. 21(3): p. 568–70.

[84] Marmont, A.M., et al., *Allogeneic bone marrow transplantation (BMT) for refractory Behcet's disease with severe CNS involvement.* Bone Marrow Transplant, 2006. 37(11): p. 1061–3.

[85] Parekkadan, B. and J.M. Milwid, *Mesenchymal stem cells as therapeutics.* Annu Rev Biomed Eng, 2010. 12: p. 87–117.

[86] Dasari, V.R., K.K. Veeravalli, and D.H. Dinh, *Mesenchymal stem cells in the treatment of spinal cord injuries: A review.* World J Stem Cells, 2014. 6(2): p. 120–33.

[87] Vawda, R. and M.G. Fehlings, *Mesenchymal cells in the treatment of spinal cord injury: current & future perspectives.* Curr Stem Cell Res Ther, 2013. 8(1): p. 25–38.

[88] White, S.V., et al., *Intravenous transplantation of mesenchymal progenitors distribute solely to the lungs and improve outcomes in cervical spinal cord injury.* Stem Cells, 2016. DOI: 10.1002/STEM.2364

[89] Lee, R.H., et al., *Intravenous hMSCs improve myocardial infarction in mice because cells embolized in lung are activated to secrete the anti-inflammatory protein TSG-6.* Cell Stem Cell, 2009. 5(1): p. 54–63.

[90] Zangi, L., et al., *Direct imaging of immune rejection and memory induction by allogeneic mesenchymal stromal cells.* Stem Cells, 2009. 27(11): p. 2865–74.

[91] Paul, C., et al., *Grafting of human bone marrow stromal cells into spinal cord injury: a comparison of delivery methods.* Spine (Phila Pa 1976), 2009. 34(4): p. 328–34.

[92] Saito, F., et al., *Spinal cord injury treatment with intrathecal autologous bone marrow stromal cell transplantation: the first clinical trial case report.* J Trauma, 2008. 64(1): p. 53–9.

[93] Kopen, G.C., D.J. Prockop, and D.G. Phinney, *Marrow stromal cells migrate throughout forebrain and cerebellum, and they differentiate into astrocytes after injection into neonatal mouse brains.* Proc Natl Acad Sci U S A, 1999. 96(19): p. 10711–6.

[94] Hofstetter, C.P., et al., *Marrow stromal cells form guiding strands in the injured spinal cord and promote recovery.* Proc Natl Acad Sci U S A, 2002. 99(4): p. 2199–204.

[95] Martinez, A.M., et al., *Neurotrauma and mesenchymal stem cells treatment: from experimental studies to clinical trials.* World J Stem Cells, 2014. 6(2): p. 179–94.

[96] Uccelli, A., et al., *Neuroprotective features of mesenchymal stem cells.* Best Pract Res Clin Haematol, 2011. 24(1): p. 59–64.

[97] Abrams, M.B., et al., *Multipotent mesenchymal stromal cells attenuate chronic inflammation and injury-induced sensitivity to mechanical stimuli in experimental spinal cord injury.* Restor Neurol Neurosci, 2009. 27(4): p. 307–21.

[98] Lu, P., et al., *Combinatorial therapy with neurotrophins and cAMP promotes axonal regeneration beyond sites of spinal cord injury.* J Neurosci, 2004. 24(28): p. 6402–9.

[99] Lu, P., L.L. Jones, and M.H. Tuszynski, *BDNF-expressing marrow stromal cells support extensive axonal growth at sites of spinal cord injury.* Exp Neurol, 2005. 191(2): p. 344–60.

[100] Lu, P., L.L. Jones, and M.H. Tuszynski, *Axon regeneration through scars and into sites of chronic spinal cord injury.* Exp Neurol, 2007. 203(1): p. 8–21.

[101] Novikova, L.N., et al., *Neuroprotective and growth-promoting effects of bone marrow stromal cells after cervical spinal cord injury in adult rats.* Cytotherapy, 2011. 13(7): p. 873–87.

[102] Sandner, B., et al., *Bone morphogenetic proteins prevent bone marrow stromal cell-mediated oligodendroglial differentiation of transplanted adult neural progenitor cells in the injured spinal cord.* Stem Cell Res, 2013. 11(2): p. 758–71.

[103] Bhanot, Y., et al., *Autologous mesenchymal stem cells in chronic spinal cord injury.* Br J Neurosurg, 2011. 25(4): p. 516–22.

[104] Goldschlager, T., et al., *Cervical motion preservation using mesenchymal progenitor cells and pentosan polysulfate, a novel chondrogenic agent: preliminary study in an ovine model.* Neurosurg Focus, 2010. 28(6): p. E4.

[105] Zuk, P.A., et al., *Multilineage cells from human adipose tissue: implications for cell-based therapies.* Tissue Eng, 2001. 7(2): p. 211–28.

[106] Kolar, M.K., et al., *The therapeutic effects of human adipose-derived stem cells in a rat cervical spinal cord injury model.* Stem Cells Dev, 2014. 23(14): p. 1659–74.

[107] Saporta, S., et al., *Human umbilical cord blood stem cells infusion in spinal cord injury: engraftment and beneficial influence on behavior.* J Hematother Stem Cell Res, 2003. 12(3): p. 271–8.

[108] Dasari, V.R., et al., *Axonal remyelination by cord blood stem cells after spinal cord injury.* J Neurotrauma, 2007. 24(2): p. 391–410.

[109] Park, D.H., et al., *Transplantation of umbilical cord blood stem cells for treating spinal cord injury.* Stem Cell Rev, 2011. 7(1): p. 181–94.

[110] Wei, L., et al., *Multiple injections of human umbilical cord-derived mesenchymal stromal cells through the tail vein improve microcirculation and the microenvironment in a rat model of radiation myelopathy.* J Transl Med, 2014. 12: p. 246.

[111] Tetzlaff, W., et al., *A systematic review of cellular transplantation therapies for spinal cord injury.* J Neurotrauma, 2011. 28(8): p. 1611–82.

[112] Tsuji, O., et al., *Cell therapy for spinal cord injury by neural stem/progenitor cells derived from iPS/ES cells.* Neurotherapeutics, 2011. 8(4): p. 668–76.

[113] Willerth, S.M., *Neural tissue engineering using embryonic and induced pluripotent stem cells.* Stem Cell Res Ther, 2011. 2(2): p. 17.

[114] Evans, M.J. and M.H. Kaufman, *Establishment in culture of pluripotential cells from mouse embryos.* Nature, 1981. 292(5819): p. 154–6.

[115] Martin, G.R., *Isolation of a pluripotent cell line from early mouse embryos cultured in medium conditioned by teratocarcinoma stem cells.* Proc Natl Acad Sci U S A, 1981. 78(12): p. 7634–8.

[116] Thomson, J.A., et al., *Embryonic stem cell lines derived from human blastocysts.* Science, 1998. 282(5391): p. 1145–7.

[117] Pera, M.F. and A.O. Trounson, *Human embryonic stem cells: prospects for development.* Development, 2004. 131(22): p. 5515–25.

[118] Braam, S.R., et al., *Feeder-free culture of human embryonic stem cells in conditioned medium for efficient genetic modification.* Nat Protoc, 2008. 3(9): p. 1435–43.

[119] McElroy, S.L. and R.A. Reijo Pera, *Culturing human embryonic stem cells in feeder-free conditions.* CSH Protoc, 2008. 2008: doi: 10.1101/pdb.prot5044.

[120] Xu, C., et al., *Feeder-free growth of undifferentiated human embryonic stem cells.* Nat Biotech, 2001. 19(10): p. 971–974.

[121] Ko, J.Y., et al., *Human embryonic stem cell-derived neural precursors as a continuous, stable, and on-demand source for human dopamine neurons.* J Neurochem, 2007. 103(4): p. 1417–29.

[122] Richards, M., et al., *Human feeders support prolonged undifferentiated growth of human inner cell masses and embryonic stem cells.* Nat Biotechnol, 2002. 20(9): p. 933–6.

[123] Ruff, C.A., J.T. Wilcox, and M.G. Fehlings, *Cell-based transplantation strategies to promote plasticity following spinal cord injury.* Exp Neurol, 2012. 235(1): p. 78–90.

[124] Bain, G., et al., *Embryonic stem cells express neuronal properties in vitro.* Dev Biol, 1995. 168(2): p. 342–57.

[125] Kumagai, G., et al., *Roles of ES cell-derived gliogenic neural stem/progenitor cells in functional recovery after spinal cord injury.* PLoS One, 2009. 4(11): p. e7706.

[126] Salewski, R.P., et al., *Transplantation of induced pluripotent stem cell-derived neural stem cells mediate functional recovery following thoracic spinal cord injury through remyelination of axons.* Stem Cells Transl Med, 2015. 4(7): p. 743–54.

[127] Cloutier, F., et al., *Transplantation of human embryonic stem cell-derived oligodendrocyte progenitors into rat spinal cord injuries does not cause harm.* Regen Med, 2006. 1(4): p. 469–79.

[128] Faulkner, J. and H.S. Keirstead, *Human embryonic stem cell-derived oligodendrocyte progenitors for the treatment of spinal cord injury.* Transpl Immunol, 2005. 15(2): p. 131–42.

[129] Liu, S., et al., *Embryonic stem cells differentiate into oligodendrocytes and myelinate in culture and after spinal cord transplantation.* Proc Natl Acad Sci U S A, 2000. 97(11): p. 6126–31.

[130] Nistor, G., et al., *Derivation of high purity neuronal progenitors from human embryonic stem cells.* PLoS One, 2011. 6(6): p. e20692.

[131] Sharp, J., et al., *Derivation of oligodendrocyte progenitor cells from human embryonic stem cells.* Methods Mol Biol, 2011. 767: p. 399–409.

[132] Wichterle, H., et al., *Directed differentiation of embryonic stem cells into motor neurons.* Cell, 2002. 110(3): p. 385–97.

[133] Peljto, M., et al., *Functional diversity of ESC-derived motor neuron subtypes revealed through intraspinal transplantation.* Cell Stem Cell, 2010. 7(3): p. 355–66.

[134] Wyatt, T.J., et al., *Human motor neuron progenitor transplantation leads to endogenous neuronal sparing in 3 models of motor neuron loss.* Stem Cells Int, 2011. 2011: p. 207230.

[135] Johnson, P.J., et al., *Tissue-engineered fibrin scaffolds containing neural progenitors enhance functional recovery in a subacute model of SCI.* Soft Matter, 2010. 6(20): p. 5127–5137.

[136] McCreedy, D.A., et al., *A new method for generating high purity motoneurons from mouse embryonic stem cells.* Biotechnol Bioeng, 2014. 111(10): p. 2041–55.

[137] McCreedy, D.A., et al., *Transgenic enrichment of mouse embryonic stem cell-derived progenitor motor neurons.* Stem Cell Res, 2012. 8(3): p. 368–78.

[138] McCreedy, D.A., et al., *Survival, differentiation, and migration of high-purity mouse embryonic stem cell-derived progenitor motor neurons in fibrin scaffolds after sub-acute spinal cord injury.* Biomater Sci, 2014. 2(11): p. 1672–82.

[139] Ideguchi, M., et al., *Murine embryonic stem cell-derived pyramidal neurons integrate into the cerebral cortex and appropriately project axons to subcortical targets.* J Neurosci, 2010. 30(3): p. 894–904.

[140] Sharp, J., et al., *Human embryonic stem cell-derived oligodendrocyte progenitor cell transplants improve recovery after cervical spinal cord injury.* Stem Cells, 2010. 28(1): p. 152–63.

[141] Hatch, M.N., G. Nistor, and H.S. Keirstead, *Derivation of high-purity oligodendroglial progenitors.* Methods Mol Biol, 2009. 549: p. 59–75.

[142] Nistor, G.I., et al., *Human embryonic stem cells differentiate into oligodendrocytes in high purity and myelinate after spinal cord transplantation.* Glia, 2005. 49(3): p. 385–96.

[143] Baker, M., *Stem-cell pioneer bows out.* Nature, 2011. 479(7374): p. 459.

[144] Hayden, E.C., *Funding windfall rescues abandoned stem-cell trial.* Nature, 2014. 510(7503): p. 18.

[145] Sun, Y., et al., *Transplantation of oligodendrocyte precursor cells improves locomotion deficits in rats with spinal cord irradiation injury.* PLoS One, 2013. 8(2): p. e57534.

[146] Du, Z.W., et al., *Induced expression of Olig2 is sufficient for oligodendrocyte specification but not for motoneuron specification and astrocyte repression.* Mol Cell Neurosci, 2006. 33(4): p. 371–80.

[147] Rossi, S.L., et al., *Histological and functional benefit following transplantation of motor neuron progenitors to the injured rat spinal cord.* PLoS One, 2010. 5(7): p. e11852.

[148] Diener, P.S. and B.S. Bregman, *Fetal spinal cord transplants support growth of supraspinal and segmental projections after cervical spinal cord hemisection in the neonatal rat.* J Neurosci, 1998. 18(2): p. 779–93.

[149] Lepore, A.C., et al., *Neural precursor cells can be delivered into the injured cervical spinal cord by intrathecal injection at the lumbar cord.* Brain Res, 2005. 1045(1–2): p. 206–16.

[150] Lepore, A.C. and I. Fischer, *Lineage-restricted neural precursors survive, migrate, and differentiate following transplantation into the injured adult spinal cord.* Exp Neurol, 2005. 194(1): p. 230–42.

[151] Lu, P., et al., *Long-distance growth and connectivity of neural stem cells after severe spinal cord injury.* Cell, 2012. 150(6): p. 1264–73.

[152] Giovanini, M.A., et al., *Characteristics of human fetal spinal cord grafts in the adult rat spinal cord: influences of lesion and grafting conditions.* Exp Neurol, 1997. 148(2): p. 523–43.

[153] Reier, P.J., et al., *Workshop on intraspinal transplantation and clinical application.* J Neurotrauma, 1994. 11(4): p. 369–77.

[154] Reier, P.J., et al., *Fetal cell grafts into resection and contusion/compression injuries of the rat and cat spinal cord.* Exp Neurol, 1992. 115(1): p. 177–88.

[155] Anderson, D.K., D.R. Howland, and P.J. Reier, *Fetal neural grafts and repair of the injured spinal cord.* Brain Pathol, 1995. 5(4): p. 451–57.

[156] Anderson, D.K., et al., *Delayed grafting of fetal CNS tissue into chronic compression lesions of the adult cat spinal cord.* Restor Neurol Neurosci, 1991. 2(4): p. 309–25.

[157] Reier, P.J., *Neural tissue grafts and repair of the injured spinal cord.* Neuropathol Appl Neurobiol, 1985. 11(2): p. 81–104.

[158] Diener, P.S. and B.S. Bregman, *Fetal spinal cord transplants support the development of target reaching and coordinated postural adjustments after neonatal cervical spinal cord injury.* J Neurosci, 1998. 18(2): p. 763–78.

[159] StemCells, Inc., *Study of human central nervous system (CNS) stem cell transplantation in cervical spinal cord injury. In: ClinicalTrials.gov [Internet]*, 2000-2015, National Library of Medicine (US): Bethesda. MD, *Jan 16. Available from: https://clinicaltrials.gov/ct2/show/ NCT02163876 NLM Indentifier: NCT02163876.*

[160] Cizkova, D., et al., *Functional recovery in rats with ischemic paraplegia after spinal grafting of human spinal stem cells.* Neuroscience, 2007. 147(2): p. 546–60.

[161] van Gorp, S., et al., *Amelioration of motor/sensory dysfunction and spasticity in a rat model of acute lumbar spinal cord injury by human neural stem cell transplantation.* Stem Cell Res Ther, 2013. 4(3): p. 57.

[162] Salewski, R.P., et al., *Transplantation of neural stem cells clonally derived from embryonic stem cells promotes recovery after murine spinal cord injury.* Stem Cells Dev, 2015. 24(1): p. 36–50.

[163] Miura, K., et al., *Variation in the safety of induced pluripotent stem cell lines.* Nat Biotechnol, 2009. 27(8): p. 743–5.

[164] Takahashi, K., et al., *Induction of pluripotent stem cells from adult human fibroblasts by defined factors.* Cell, 2007. 131(5): p. 861–72.

[165] Takahashi, K. and S. Yamanaka, *Induction of pluripotent stem cells from mouse embryonic and adult fibroblast cultures by defined factors.* Cell, 2006. 126(4): p. 663–76.

[166] Yamanaka, Shinya. "Patient-specific pluripotent stem cells become even more accessible." *Cell Stem Cell* 7.1 (2010): 1–2.

[167] Fusaki, Noemi, et al. "Efficient induction of transgene-free human pluripotent stem cells using a vector based on Sendai virus, an RNA virus that does not integrate into the host genome." *Proceedings of the Japan Academy, Series B* 85.8 (2009): 348–362.

[168] Nori, Satoshi, et al. "Long-term safety issues of iPSC-based cell therapy in a spinal cord injury model: oncogenic transformation with epithelial-mesenchymal transition." *Stem cell reports* 4.3 (2015): 360–373.

[169] Zhou, Hongyan, et al. "Generation of induced pluripotent stem cells using recombinant proteins." *Cell stem cell* 4.5 (2009): 381–384.

[170] Warren, Luigi, et al. "Highly efficient reprogramming to pluripotency and directed differentiation of human cells with synthetic modified mRNA." *Cell stem cell* 7.5 (2010): 618–630.

[171] Rao, Mahendra S., and Nasir Malik. "Assessing iPSC reprogramming methods for their suitability in translational medicine." *Journal of cellular biochemistry* 113.10 (2012): 3061–3068.

[172] Brennand, K.J., et al., *Modeling psychiatric disorders at the cellular and network levels.* Mol Psychiatry, 2012. 17(12): p. 1239–53.

[173]   Han, S.S., L.A. Williams, and K.C. Eggan, *Constructing and deconstructing stem cell models of neurological disease.* Neuron, 2011. 70(4): p. 626–44.

[174]   Marchetto, M.C. and F.H. Gage, *Modeling brain disease in a dish: really?* Cell Stem Cell, 2012. 10(6): p. 642–5.

[175]   Guo, J., et al., *Contribution of mouse embryonic stem cells and induced pluripotent stem cells to chimeras through injection and coculture of embryos.* Stem Cells Int, 2014. 2014: p. 409021.

[176]   Parmar, M. and A. Bjorklund, *Generation of transplantable striatal projection neurons from human ESCs.* Cell Stem Cell, 2012. 10(4): p. 349–50.

[177]   Barker, R.A., *Developing stem cell therapies for Parkinson's disease: waiting until the time is right.* Cell Stem Cell, 2014. 15(5): p. 539–42.

[178]   Ambasudhan, R., et al., *Direct reprogramming of adult human fibroblasts to functional neurons under defined conditions.* Cell Stem Cell, 2011. 9(2): p. 113–8.

[179]   Vierbuchen, T., et al., *Direct conversion of fibroblasts to functional neurons by defined factors.* Nature, 2010. 463(7284): p. 1035–41.

[180]   Zhang, Y., et al., *Rapid single-step induction of functional neurons from human pluripotent stem cells.* Neuron, 2013. 78(5): p. 785–98.

[181]   Molyneaux, B.J., et al., *Neuronal subtype specification in the cerebral cortex.* Nat Rev Neurosci, 2007. 8(6): p. 427–37.

[182]   Arlotta, P., et al., *Neuronal subtype-specific genes that control corticospinal motor neuron development in vivo.* Neuron, 2005. 45(2): p. 207–21.

[183]   Byers, B., et al., *SNCA triplication Parkinson's patient's iPSC-derived DA neurons accumulate alpha-synuclein and are susceptible to oxidative stress.* PLoS One, 2011. 6(11): p. e26159.

[184]   Nguyen, H.N., et al., *LRRK2 mutant iPSC-derived DA neurons demonstrate increased susceptibility to oxidative stress.* Cell Stem Cell, 2011. 8(3): p. 267–80.

[185]   Dolmetsch, R. and D.H. Geschwind, *The human brain in a dish: the promise of iPSC-derived neurons.* Cell, 2011. 145(6): p. 831–4.

[186]   Pera, M.F., *Stem cells: the dark side of induced pluripotency.* Nature, 2011. 471(7336): p. 46–7.

[187]   Boulting, G.L., et al., *A functionally characterized test set of human induced pluripotent stem cells.* Nat Biotechnol, 2011. 29(3): p. 279–86.

[188]   Brennand, K.J. and F.H. Gage, *Concise review: the promise of human induced pluripotent stem cell-based studies of schizophrenia.* Stem Cells, 2011. 29(12): p. 1915–22.

[189]   Brennand, K.J., et al., *Modelling schizophrenia using human induced pluripotent stem cells.* Nature, 2011. 473(7346): p. 221–5.

[190] Faravelli, I., et al., *iPSC-based models to unravel key pathogenetic processes underlying motor neuron disease development.* J Clin Med, 2014. 3(4): p. 1124–45.

[191] Hirami, Y., et al., *Generation of retinal cells from mouse and human induced pluripotent stem cells.* Neurosci Lett, 2009. 458(3): p. 126–31.

[192] Hodgetts, S.I., M. Edel, and A.R. Harvey, *The state of play with iPSCs and spinal cord injury models.* J Clin Med, 2015. 4(1): p. 193–203.

[193] Hu, B.Y., et al., *Neural differentiation of human induced pluripotent stem cells follows developmental principles but with variable potency.* Proc Natl Acad Sci U S A, 2010. 107(9): p. 4335–40.

[194] Kim, J., et al., *Reprogramming of postnatal neurons into induced pluripotent stem cells by defined factors.* Stem Cells, 2011. 29(6): p. 992–1000.

[195] Kim, J.E., et al., *Investigating synapse formation and function using human pluripotent stem cell-derived neurons.* Proc Natl Acad Sci U S A, 2011. 108(7): p. 3005–10.

[196] Marchetto, M.C., et al., *A model for neural development and treatment of Rett syndrome using human induced pluripotent stem cells.* Cell, 2010. 143(4): p. 527–39.

[197] Zeng, H., et al., *Specification of region-specific neurons including forebrain glutamatergic neurons from human induced pluripotent stem cells.* PLoS One, 2010. 5(7): p. e11853.

[198] Kim, J., et al., *Direct reprogramming of mouse fibroblasts to neural progenitors.* Proc Natl Acad Sci U S A, 2011. 108(19): p. 7838–43.

[199] Marchetto, M.C., B. Winner, and F.H. Gage, *Pluripotent stem cells in neurodegenerative and neurodevelopmental diseases.* Hum Mol Genet, 2010. 19(R1): p. R71–6.

[200] Krencik, R. and S.C. Zhang, *Directed differentiation of functional astroglial subtypes from human pluripotent stem cells.* Nat Protoc, 2011. 6(11): p. 1710–7.

[201] Yang, N., et al., *Generation of oligodendroglial cells by direct lineage conversion.* Nat Biotechnol, 2013. 31(5): p. 434–9.

[202] All, A.H., et al., *Human embryonic stem cell-derived oligodendrocyte progenitors aid in functional recovery of sensory pathways following contusive spinal cord injury.* PLoS One, 2012. 7(10): p. e47645.

[203] Hayashi, K., et al., *Increase of sensitivity to mechanical stimulus after transplantation of murine induced pluripotent stem cell-derived astrocytes in a rat spinal cord injury model.* J Neurosurg Spine, 2011. 15(6): p. 582–93.

[204] Fujimoto, Y., et al., *Treatment of a mouse model of spinal cord injury by transplantation of human induced pluripotent stem cell-derived long-term self-renewing neuroepithelial-like stem cells.* Stem Cells, 2012. 30(6): p. 1163–73.

[205] Nori, S., et al., *Grafted human-induced pluripotent stem-cell-derived neurospheres promote motor functional recovery after spinal cord injury in mice.* Proc Natl Acad Sci U S A, 2011. 108(40): p. 16825–30.

[206] Tsuji, O., et al., *Therapeutic potential of appropriately evaluated safe-induced pluripotent stem cells for spinal cord injury.* Proc Natl Acad Sci U S A, 2010. 107(28): p. 12704–9.

[207] Li, K., et al., *Human iPS cell-derived astrocyte transplants preserve respiratory function after spinal cord injury.* Exp Neurol, 2015. 271: p. 479–92.

[208] Lu, P., et al., *Long-distance axonal growth from human induced pluripotent stem cells after spinal cord injury.* Neuron, 2014. 83(4): p. 789–96.

[209] Nutt, S.E., et al., *Caudalized human iPSC-derived neural progenitor cells produce neurons and glia but fail to restore function in an early chronic spinal cord injury model.* Exp Neurol, 2013. 248: p. 491–503.

[210] Kobayashi, Y., et al., *Pre-evaluated safe human iPSC-derived neural stem cells promote functional recovery after spinal cord injury in common marmoset without tumorigenicity.* PLoS One, 2012. 7(12): p. e52787.

4

Role of JAK-STAT Signalling on Motor Function Recovery after Spinal Cord Injury

Victor S. Tapia and Juan Larrain

Abstract

JAK-STAT signalling is a main transduction pathway of cytokines and growth factors, which is involved in several biological processes including cell proliferation, cell differentiation, axon regeneration, apoptosis and inflammation. After spinal cord injury several cytokines activate the JAK-STAT pathway, thereby modulating several cell responses. In this chapter we discuss how regulation of this signalling pathway could improve motor recovery after injury by modulation of axon regeneration, neuroprotection, glial scar formation, demyelination and inflammatory response. Studies with gene over-expression, gene deletion and *in vitro* approaches will be discussed for understanding the cell-specific response to JAK-STAT signalling, with a focus on preclinical treatment with IL6-family cytokines, hematopoietic cytokines and IL10.

Keywords: cytokine, JAK-STAT, STAT3, axon regeneration, glial scar, inflammation

1. Introduction

Worldwide, an estimate of 180,000 cases of spinal cord injuries (SCI) occur yearly [1]. SCI results in the complete or partial loss of motor and sensory functions below the lesion site. This type of injury causes irreversible paralysis, chronic pain, loss of bladder, bowel and sexual function, amongst others dysfunctions, impairing quality and increasing the cost of life [2, 3].

The pathology of SCI in mammals starts with an acute phase during the first days of injury, which includes massive cell death and inflammatory response. The acute response is followed by a second phase during the first week after injury consisting of tissue replacement, where the loss of cells is replaced by a glial scar. After the second week it finalizes with a third phase which continues for months involving chronic tissue remodelling, remyelination and circuit remodelling [4]. Although some spontaneous repair after SCI has been described in mammals including humans, it contributes poorly to motor and functional recovery. Progenitor cells proliferate and differentiate but mostly to glial cells while no neurogenesis occurs [5, 6]. Besides there is only a partial axon regeneration and circuit remodelling response that contribute to a limited compensatory recovery [2].

Several reviews have been published describing growth factors and cytokines that regulate cell response in SCI [2, 7, 8]. Advancements using these factors to improve spinal cord repair are being made, and preclinical treatments have been achieved by local delivery of growth factors and by physiological delivery with i.v. or i.p. injections (intravenous or intraperitoneal, respectively) [2]. Between the plethora of signalling pathways activated in response to tissue injury, the JAK-STAT signalling pathway is one of the main pathways that has been extensively studied because of its broad effect on the response to injury. In this chapter, we discuss the activation and role of JAK-STAT signalling in response to SCI and studies focused on modulating JAK-STAT to improve motor recovery. First, we briefly describe the JAK-STAT pathway components, followed by a discussion of its role in different cellular processes including: axonal regeneration, neuroprotection, glial response and its effects on the inflammatory response.

2. JAK-STAT signalling pathway

The JAK-STAT signalling pathway is involved in transmitting information from the extracellular milieu to gene promoters in the nucleus. The basic components of the JAK-STAT pathway are depicted in **Figure 1**. Several cytokines, growth factors and even hormones signal through the JAK-STAT pathway. Currently, there are 38 protein ligands and 36 cell surface receptor combinations have been described [9]. Besides the several combinations of protein ligands and receptor complexes, in mammals there are four JAK (Janus kinase) tyrosine kinases: JAK1, JAK2, JAK3 and Tyk2 (Non-receptor tyrosine-protein kinase TYK2); and seven STAT (Signal transducer and activator of transcription) transcription factors: STAT1, STAT2, STAT3, STAT4, STAT5a, STAT5b and STAT6 [9].

Activation of the JAK-STAT pathway begins after ligand binding to the receptor subunits, which forms homodimers, heterodimers or heteromultimers depending on the family receptor (**Table 1** presents ligands and receptors related to SCI). After multimerization, intracellular transduction is initiated through the recruitment of JAK kinases. JAKs phosphorylate receptor subunits and STAT transcription factors. After tyrosine phosphorylation, cytosolic STATs dimerize and are translocated to the nucleus to bind specific DNA regulatory sequences and regulate gene expression [10].

The JAK-STAT signalling pathway has different negative inhibitors. The most important inhibitor for preclinical studies is the classical negative feedback loop of suppressor of cytokine signalling (SOCS) proteins, which are target genes for STATs proteins and switch off JAK proteins. Over-expression or deletion of SOCS3, one of the eight mammalian SOCS proteins, has been extensively used to modulate endogenous pathway activation [11–13].

Although it will not be discussed in this chapter, it has to be considered that ligands binding to receptor complexes also activate other intracellular signalling cascades besides the JAK-STAT pathway [10]. Phosphorylation of receptors induces activation of ERK1/2 and AKT pathways. Moreover, STATs can also be activated independently to the canonical JAK-STAT signalling pathway. Growth factor activation of RTKs (receptor tyrosine kinases) and NRTKs (non-receptor tyrosine kinases) can activate STATs. Hormone and chemokine binding to G protein–coupled receptors can also activate JAKs proteins to phosphorylate STATs [10].

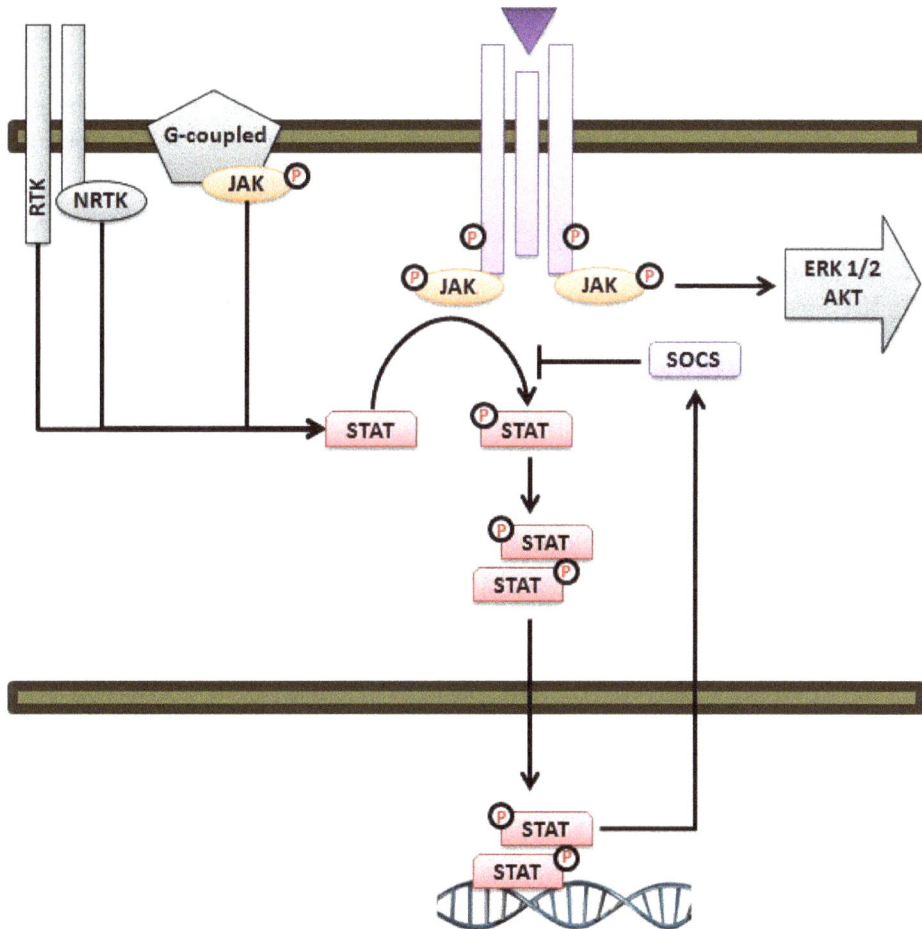

Figure 1. Basic components of the JAK-STAT signaling pathway. After binding of cytokines, receptors multimerize (violet boxes) recruiting to the membrane and activating JAK kinases (orange boxes) that initiate substrate phosphorylation (letter P). STAT transcription factors (pink boxes) are phosphorylated, dimerized and transported to the nucleus. STAT dimers regulate gene transcription. Among others, a classic target is SOCS that forms a negative feedback loop inhibiting JAK function. Alternative signaling pathways (grey boxes) for JAK-STAT are JAK-receptor complex activation of ERK1/2 and AKT pathways; STATs phosphorylation by RTKs, NRTKs or JAKs associated to G-coupled protein receptors.

3. JAK-STAT pathway activation in response to SCI

3.1. Cytokine expression in response to SCI

Before discussing the role of the JAK-STAT pathway in motor recovery, we will discuss the endogenous expression of cytokines and activation of STAT proteins in response to SCI. The upregulation of the IL6 family cytokines, IL6 (Interleukin 6), LIF (Leukemia inhibitory factor), OSM (Oncostatin M), IL11 (Interleukin 11) and CNTF (Ciliary neurotrophic factor) have been well characterized in response to SCI. Early IL6 and LIF upregulation has been detected in the acute phase after SCI, with a peak of expression around 6–12 hpi (hours post-injury) and basal levels at 4 dpi (days post-injury) [14, 15]. Different neural cell types contribute to IL6 and LIF expression. It has been shown that IL6 has a broad cell type expression, being detected in neurons, astrocytes and macrophages, while LIF is mainly expressed in meningeal astrocytes [14]. IL6 mRNA expression correlates with IL6 protein levels analyzed in another study, which detected an increase in IL6 concentration from 3 hours to 3 dpi [16]. In these studies the upregulation of cytokines occurs in the surrounding area of the lesion site, around 1 or 2 mm from the epicentre.

Early upregulation of OSM is also detected after SCI, with a strong peak at 6 hpi, but on the contrary to IL6 and LIF, upregulation of OSM is still detected until 1 mpi (months post-injury) [15]. IL11 and CNTF protein upregulation has also been detected after the acute phase. A steady increase in protein levels has been detected during the first week of injury for IL11 and during the first month for CNTF. In both cases no later times were analyzed to determine when the cytokines reached basal levels, therefore there is a possibility that they had an extended upregulation [17, 18]. IL11 cell expression has not been analyzed; on the contrary, it has been shown that CNTF has a chronic expression in glial cell types after spinal cord injury. CNTF has been detected in oligodendrocytes during the first month and in astrocytes up to 4 mpi [18, 19]. This chronic expression of CNTF is more spatially restricted than the early expressed cytokines IL6 and LIF, being detected only in the lesion borders [19].

Cytokine family	Cytokine	Receptors	JAKs	STATs	Endogenous levels, preclinical or clinical trials
IL6	IL6	Gp130 – IL6R	Jak1	STAT1-3	U/P
	LIF	Gp130 – LIFR	Jak2	STAT3	U/P
	CNTF	Gp130 – LIFR – CNTFR	Tyk2	STAT3	U/P
	IL11	Gp130 – IL11R		STAT3	U
	OSM	Gp130 –		STAT3	U/P

Cytokine family	Cytokine	Receptors	JAKs	STATs	Endogenous levels, preclinical or clinical trials
		LIFR			
Hematopoietic	G-CSF	CSF3R	Jak2	STAT3	P/C
	GM-CSF	CSF2Ra – βcR	Jak2	STAT5a/b	P/C
	EPO	EpoR or EpoR-βcR	Jak2	STAT5a/b	P/C
IL10	IL10	IL10Rα – IL10Rβ	Jak1 – Tyk2	STAT1-3	P

Table 1. JAK-STAT ligands, receptors and transducers involved in spinal cord injury. Cytokines are shown with associated receptors and JAK-STAT components. It is shown if cytokines are up-regulated in response to SCI (U) or if they have been used in preclinical (P) or clinical (C) studies for spinal cord recovery.

3.2. JAK-STAT signalling in response to SCI

In concordance with the upregulation of cytokines in response to SCI, several studies have characterized JAK-STAT pathway activation in spinal cord cells. Consistent with the transient increase of IL6 concentration, in the same study it was detected an increase in gp130 dimerization and JAK1 phosphorylation [16]. As expected for the activation of the gp130/JAK1 axis, STAT1 and STAT3 are phosphorylated in response to SCI. pSTAT1 has an acute increase which reach basal levels at 2 dpi [20]. On the contrary, pSTAT3 has an extended increase which differs between studies. An increase in pSTAT3 has been detected up to 7 dpi in some studies [12, 16], while in another no basal levels were reached even after 2 weeks post-injury (wpi) [21]. Nevertheless, all studies agree that STAT3 has a longer activation than STAT1. Together with the temporal difference, protein localization suggests that STAT3 has a more prominent role in regulating gene expression than STAT1 in cell response. While pSTAT3 has been detected in neuron nuclei after spinal cord injury, pSTAT1 has been only detected in the cytoplasm [16, 20].

STAT3 activation has been characterized in several spinal cord cell types. In the acute injury, nuclear pSTAT3 is observed in neurons of the anterior horns [16] and transcriptional activity is also supported by the detection of SOCS3+ neurons [21]. Nuclear pSTAT3 and SOCS3 has been also detected in microglia/macrophage during the acute phase of injury [16, 21] and nuclear pSTAT3 in oligodendrocytes and astrocytes during the first week near the lesion site [12, 22]. Due to a prominent role in glial scar formation, spatial STAT3 activation on astrocytes has also been highly defined. It has been determined that during the first week pSTAT3+ astrocytes appear at the border of the lesion with elevated predominance on the first 500 μm near the injury [12, 22].

After the first week of injury, contusion models show chronic pSTAT3 signalling in glial cell types located in the lesion borders. pSTAT3 has been detected in oligodendrocyte precursor cells (OPCs) and oligodendrocytes at 2 wpi [18, 19]. This activation decreases from 1 to 5 wpi, but at that time is still higher than on uninjured spinal cords [19]. pSTAT3+ astrocytes have been detected even further, at 12 wpi in the lesion borders [19].

4. Role of JAK-STAT in axon regeneration and collateral sprouting

To recover motor function after SCI, new connections have to be established after neuron death and axon degeneration [2]. These circuits can be established by two different cellular responses that should not be confused: Axon regeneration is the process where axons from severed neurons regrow from the injured tip or from a lateral growth distant to the injury (**Figure 2a-b**). On the contrary, collateral sprouting is a compensatory growth from undamaged axons initiated in response to injury (**Figure 2c**) [23].

While there is limited axon regeneration through the lesion area in response to complete SCI (**Figure 2a**), there is a compensatory remodelling on brain and spinal circuits when the spinal

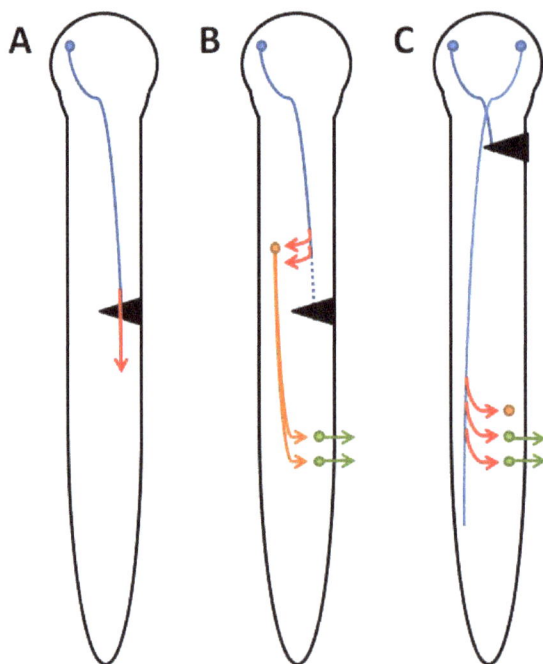

Figure 2. Axonal regeneration and collateral sprouting in spinal cord injury. Models used to evaluate axon regeneration and circuit remodeling, showing corticospinal tract (CST, in blue) as an example. Remodeling can be evaluated by axonal regeneration or collateral sprouting (both in red arrows) and new innervations can be connected to propiospinal neurons (PSNs, interneurons in orange) or motor neurons (in green). CNS injury is indicated as a darkened triangle in every model. **A**, In SCI models (usually contusion and hemisection) axonal regeneration of injured CSTs can be evaluated through and beyond the lesion area. **B**, in a hemisection model, innervation of new targets by injured CSTs can be evaluated. Regenerative axons from CSTs can innervate PSNs, which then connect to denervated motoneurons. **C**, in a unilateral pyramidotomy injury paradigm, collateral sprouting of uninjured CSTs to denervated PSNs and motor neurons can be measured. Anterograde, retrograde or retrograde trans-synaptic labelling are used depending of the injury model.

cord lesion is incomplete [2]. The corticospinal tract (CST) has been used as a model to study this recovery process. CST starts in the motor cortex and connects to spinal motor neurons, controlling voluntary motor function [23]. After spinal cord injury, CST circuit remodelling can be achieved by axon regeneration innervating long descendent interneurons that increase connection to motoneurons (**Figure 2b**) [24] or by collateral sprouting of uninjured axons to denervated motoneurons (**Figure 2c**) [25]. In this section we will discuss the role of JAK-STAT pathway on the promotion of axon regeneration and collateral sprouting after SCI. Briefly, we will discuss the results involving dorsal root ganglion (DRG) and optic nerve injury, to follow with studies of axon growth and collateral sprouting of the CSTs after SCI.

4.1. Role of JAK-STAT pathway in axon regeneration in SCI and other nerve injury models

4.1.1. Axon regeneration after dorsal root ganglion or optic nerve axotomy

The DRG model has been useful to study axon regeneration due to regenerative and non-regenerative branches. Sensory neurons from DRG target peripheral tissue with branches (i.e. sciatic nerve) that regenerate after axotomy. On the contrary, DRG neurons also target the dorsal column of the spinal cord, which do not regenerate after injury. This difference in the regenerative capacity has been partially related to the JAK-STAT pathway activation by studies on cytokine deficient mice, but conclusive results have been obtained in a study assessing the role of STAT3 in axon regeneration. While STAT3 deletion reduced axon growth of the severed sciatic nerve, STAT3 viral over-expression in the DRG improves axon regeneration of the non-regenerative nerve [26].

Similar to the activation of the JAK-STAT pathway in the DRG model, axon growth has been also promoted in the non-regenerative optic nerve. JAK-STAT activation by CNTF treatment or deletion of the SOCS3 negative feedback improved axon regeneration in optic nerve injury [11]. The studies in both injury models demonstrate that the JAK-STAT pathway, specifically the axis of STAT3/SOCS3, promotes axon regeneration. Therefore, a possible mechanism to improve motor recovery after SCI is through modulation of the JAK-STAT pathway to induce axon regeneration.

4.1.2. Axon regeneration after the spinal cord injury

A hemisection study showed that only a small subset of cortical neurons presented an increment in STAT3 and pSTAT3 levels after SCI, suggesting that on the contrary of peripheral nerves, in the spinal cord there is a lack of retrograde JAK-STAT activation [27]. As in DRG and optic nerve injury models, insufficient JAK-STAT activation could be related to the lack of axon regeneration. Several studies have shown that improvement of local extrinsic factors, such as cytokines administration, or improvement of intrinsic factors, such as the genetic modulation of the JAK-STAT pathway in neurons, improves axon regeneration after SCI, suggesting that modulation of JAK-STAT can be a bona fide target for designing novel therapies for spinal cord repair.

Administration of CNTF, G-CSF (granulocyte-colony stimulating factor), IL6 and LIF by intrathecal or i.p. injections results in improved axon regeneration through the lesion site and motor recovery after SCI. CNTF intrathecal injections during the first 10 days or administration in sodium-hyaluronate particles placed in the transection site have improved functional recovery after SCI [28, 29]. Although CST axon regeneration has not been assessed in CNTF treatment, a study showed increased retrograde labelling of the rubrospinal tracts [28]. Another study showed improved axonal sprouting through the lesion site, although it was not evaluated if these axons were from local neurons or descended from the brain [29].

Axon regeneration has also been assessed after spinal cord administration of G-CSF during 2 weeks after a hemisection [30]. CST axon regeneration was improved in the lesion site although no axon growth caudal to the injury was detected. The local G-CSF delivery also results in improvement of motor function and a similar result was observed in a transgenic mice line expressing G-CSF under the control of the MapKII promoter that is specifically activated in cortical and spinal cord neurons [30].

On the contrary to CNTF and G-CSF treatments, LIF has been administered daily by intraperitoneal injection since it is actively transported through the BBB with a mechanism involving the LIFRα receptor [31, 32]. LIF treatment for 14 days in a hemisection injury model improved the number of retrograde labelled CST and rubrospinal neurons. Improvement in motor recovery was assessed by RotaRod and Platform hang tests [32].

Although CNTF, G-CSF and LIF treatments showed an improvement in axon regeneration and motor function in rodents, in these studies the activation of the JAK-STAT pathway in cortical neurons was not assessed. Besides, these studies cannot distinguish if the improvement in axon regeneration and functional recovery is due to the modulation of the intrinsic program of cortical neurons or due to the modulation of other spinal cord cell types. Contrary to these studies, local IL6 administration has been shown to activate the JAK-STAT pathway in spinal and cortical neurons [33, 34]. IL6 intrathecal administration during the first week after a hemisection injury increased pSTAT3 levels in the spinal cord and in cortical neurons, while up-regulated the regeneration associated gene GAP-43 mRNA [34]. Although no motor recovery analyses were assessed, anterograde labelling showed an increase in the number of synapsin1+ CST axons near the lesion site [33].

The IL6 treatment suggests that cytokine delivery can promote the regenerative response of motoneurons by JAK-STAT pathway activation. In addition, specific STAT3 over-expression in the cortex has shown that this pathway can promote axon regeneration. After overexpression mediated by adenovirus injection in the cortex, pSTAT3 levels increased in cortical neurons and CST axonal regeneration improved through and beyond the lesion site of a hemisection [27].

4.2. Role of JAK-STAT in circuit remodelling by collateral sprouting

Although improvement in axon regeneration (**Figure 2a**) and motor recovery has been achieved by cytokine delivery, no relation has been established between the observed axon regeneration in the lesion site and the motor recovery. On the contrary, studies involving JAK-

STAT pathway and circuit remodelling by collateral sprouting (**Figure 2c**) have suggested that motor recovery is accomplished by innervation of uninjured axons to denervated motoneurons and interneurons.

Cytokine	Treatment	Cell response	Motor recovery	References
Il6	Acute by i.t.	Axon regeneration	Not assessed	[33, 34]
	Acute i.p., MR16-1	Immune modulation	Improved	[66, 84, 85]
LIF	10-14 days by i.p.	Axon regeneration Glial modulation	Improved	[32, 60, 61]
CNTF	10 days by i.p. or Hyaluronate	Axon regeneration Glial modulation	Improved	[28, 29]
	SC viral expression	Collateral sprouting	Not assessed	[13]
OSM	Gel foam	Glial modulation	Improved	[15]
G-CSF	2 weeks by i.t.	Axon regeneration Neuroprotection	Improved	[30]
	Acute by subcutaneous, i.v. or i.t.	Neuroprotection Glial modulation Immune modulation	Improved	[40, 54-57, 81]
GM-CSF	Acute by i.v., i.t. or i.p.	Glial modulation	Improved	[54, 55, 64]
EPO	Acute by i.p.	Collateral sprouting Glial modulation	Improved	[35, 58, 59]
IL10	Acute by i.p.	Glial modulation Immune modulation	Improved Not improved	[77, 78]
	SC viral expression	Neuroprotection	Improved	[48, 49]
IL12	Gel foam	Glial modulation Immune modulation	Not improved	[82]

Table 2. Pre-clinical studies with cytokine for motor recovery of SCI. Summary of JAK-STAT cytokine preclinical studies, for any cytokine it is shown administration timing and method. Time indicated as acute means a single dose at the moment of injury or daily doses from 1 to 5 dpi. Methods of administration are indicated as intrathecal (i.t.), intraperitoneal (i.p.), intravenous (i.v.) or subcutaneous injection; embedded on hyaluronate or gel foam placed in the lesion site; and by SC (spinal cord) viral expression. Contrary to the other studies, MR16-1 indicates a treatment with a neutralizing antibody against IL6 receptor.

Promotion of collateral sprouting by the hematopoietic cytokine EPO (Erythropoietin) has been assessed in a model of traumatic brain injury that results in denervation of the CST circuit. EPO i.p. injections during the acute phase resulted in increased collateral sprouting of uninjured CST fibers in the cervical and lumbar area and improved motor function [35]. Although it has not been shown that EPO activate the JAK-STAT signalling pathway in neurons, cortical viral infection has been useful to determine the role of the pathway in collateral sprouting. STAT3 viral over-expression in uninjured mice induced collateral sprouting and innervations to propiospinal neuron (PSN, a type of interneuron) [27]. This viral expression was also assessed in a unilateral pyramidotomy model, which is an injury at the level of the medulla oblongata that severs half of the CST (**Figure 2c**) and it is useful to evaluate how collateral sprouting connects to spinal neurons. In this approach it was shown that STAT3 induced collateral sprouting, innervation of PSNs and motoneurons, and improvement in motor recovery which was assessed by behavioural and electrophysiological tests [27]. Cortical SOCS3 deletion also induced collateral sprouting in the pyramidotomy paradigm [13], suggesting that an endogenous JAK-STAT pathway activation promotes circuit remodelling. After finding a transient CNTF expression in denervated neurons caudal to injury, the same study showed that combination of cortical SOCS3 deletion and spinal cord CNTF over-expression improved collateral sprouting [13].

5. Role of JAK-STAT in local neuron response

In response to SCI the number of local motor and interneurons decrease with no neurogenesis to generate new neurons [2]. To improve motor recovery, promotion of axon regeneration and collateral sprouting should be accompanied by neuroprotective strategies, since number and dendrite distribution of local spinal neurons would be beneficial for circuit remodelling. We will start this section discussing *in vitro* studies related to the neuroprotective role of the JAK-STAT pathway, following *in vivo* studies with cytokine delivery and knockdown treatments after SCI.

5.1. Role of JAK-STAT in neuron survival

At a molecular level, studies in non-neural cells have shown that STAT transcription factors have different roles in apoptosis regulation. A comparative *in vitro* study of STAT1 and STAT3 showed that while STAT1 inhibits the expression of the anti-apoptotic genes Bcl-2 and Bcl-X, STAT3 promoted their expression [36]. STAT5 proteins, which are activated by a different set of cytokines (Table 1), also promote cell survival by Bcl-X upregulation [37].

In vitro studies have shown that the neuroprotective role of JAK-STAT cytokines is partly associated to STAT3 activation and expression of anti-apoptotic genes. IL10 activated STAT3 and promoted Bcl-2 and Bcl-xl expression in embryonic spinal cord neurons [38]. IL6 and OSM cytokines also activated STAT3 and promoted anti-apoptotic gene expression in cortical neurons and neuroblastoma cells [39]. In cultured cerebellar granule neurons, G-CSF also promoted STAT3 activation while increased Bcl-2 levels [40]. It should be considered that theses cytokines also activate the AKT pathway [39, 40]. Both inhibition of the JAK and AKT pathway decreased the neuroprotective effect, suggesting that probably both pathways contribute to the anti-apoptotic response [38, 40].

Related to the previous *in vitro* studies, *in vivo* studies in CNS injury suggest a protective role of STAT3 while an opposite role for STAT1. On a focal cerebral ischemia model, it was shown that STAT1 deficient mice presented a reduced infarct size and apoptotic cell number [41]. On the contrary, on a permanent cerebral ischemia model the IL6/STAT3 axis has been associated to positive outcomes. While the neutralization with an anti-IL6R antibody resulted in decreased STAT3 activation and increased lesion area, IL6 administration reduced the lesion size [42, 43]. Although these studies indicate a neuroprotective role of STAT3, specific cell type modulation should be assessed to differentiate the direct modulation on neuron response from indirect neuroprotection by modulation of glial and inflammatory cell types. At this moment, there is only one study where specific STAT3 deletion in neurons is analyzed in an *in vivo* CNS injury model. Mice with STAT3 deletion in neurons (using the Neurofilament L promoter) showed a decrease in motoneuron number after facial nerve injury and diminished expression of anti-apoptotic genes [44].

5.2. JAK-STAT modulation of neuronal protection in SCI

G-CSF and IL10 are cytokines with several studies showing beneficial outcomes in neuroprotection, inflammatory response and motor recovery after SCI [45, 46]. It has been shown that a pro-inflammatory response is negative for neuron survival [47]; therefore, in these cytokine treatments it is difficult to differentiate a direct modulation on neuronal survival and the effect on neuro-inflammation. Since it has been shown that spinal cord neurons express G-CSF and IL10 receptors [40, 48], we will discuss a small set of studies that focused in neuroprotection and in a following section we will discuss the modulation of the immune response in SCI.

G-CSF has been locally administrated to evaluate neuroprotection in SCI. Subcutaneous G-CSF treatment during the first five days after compression improved motor recovery, decreased apoptotic neurons in the acute phase and improved neuron number in the remodelling phase (6 wpi) [40]. Other studies with intrathecal administration of G-CSF for 2 weeks, commented before for assessing axonal regeneration, also showed neuroprotective results. This long-term treatment reduced apoptotic cell number and increased Bcl-xL expression in the spinal cord [30]. Two independent IL10 viral over-expression studies also improved motor function [48, 49] and one of these studies showed decreased pro-apoptotic protein levels and increased Bcl-2 levels, resulting in a higher neuron number [48]. Although it was shown by *in vitro* studies that G-CSF and IL10 treatments activate STAT3 in spinal neurons [40, 48], it has not been demonstrated that this activation occurs on *in vivo* treatments. *In vivo* analyses of IL10 over-expression only focused in neuronal NF-κβ activation [48]. Therefore, it is an open question if these cytokines promotes neuron survival by JAK-STAT activation or by other signalling pathway, as NF-κβ gene regulation.

Although by results of cytokine treatments the role of STAT3 in neuroprotection remains inconclusive, knockdown of the inhibitory protein SOCS3 has contributed to this proposition [21]. Local over-expression of shSOCS3 diminished SOCS3 mRNA levels. This knockdown increased pSTAT3 levels in a transection model and it decreased the Bax/Bcl-2 protein ratio, while improving neuron number near the lesion site [21]. A following study of the same group showed that SOCS3 knockdown increased dendrite growth in dorsal and ventral horns near the injury site [50].

Finally, consistent with the pro-apoptotic role of STAT1 on *in vitro* studies [36], STAT1 knockdown has shown positive outcomes after SCI. Administration of STAT1 siRNA reduced STAT1 protein levels in the spinal cord. Although no analysis of neuronal survival was assessed, 1 day post-contusion the STAT1 knockdown mice had increased its Bcl-2 levels. siRNA treated mice also improved motor function assessed by BMS open-field score.

6. Role of JAK-STAT in glial response

In response to SCI, apoptosis of astrocytes and oligodendrocytes occurs in the acute phase of injury and then glial cells dynamically respond during weeks and months after injury. A glial hallmark of CNS injury is the glial scar, formed by reactive astrocytes, OPCs and meningeal cells [51]. This compact scar gathers around damaged tissue, inflammatory cells and fibroblasts. The glial scar is necessary to contain secondary injury, as disruption of the astrocyte scar with different transgenic models leads to increased cell death, demyelination and reduced functional motor recovery [12, 52, 53]. Although the glial scar is necessary for the containment of the lesion, reactive astrocytes express and secrete inhibitory molecules for axonal growth and sprouting, as chondroitin sulfate proteoglycans (CSPGs) [51]. Altogether with the glial scar formation, a demyelination process occurs during weeks after injury by oligodendrocyte apoptosis. Although mature oligodendrocytes do not proliferate to recover cell number, OPCs start to proliferate and differentiate and remyelination proceeds near the lesion area [6]. Accordingly to the glial response commented above, in this section we will discuss the following topics: Cytokine modulation of the glial response to reduce secondary damage, the regulation of reactive astrocyte and the neural stem progenitor cells (NSPCs) by the STAT3/SOCS3 axis.

6.1. Cytokines modulate glial response in SCI

Several studies with the hematopoietic and IL6-family cytokines have assessed astrocyte and oligodendrocyte responses with positive outcomes on tissue preservation and motor recovery. Acute administration of GM-CSF or G-CSF by i.p. or i.v. injections during the acute phase reduced lesion area, while increasing the spared myelin area and improving motor recovery after SCI [54–56]. Both cytokine treatments reduced NG2 levels (OPC marker) during the first week of injury [54, 55]. In one of these studies it was also shown that G-CSF up-regulated Bcl-xL and reduced apoptosis in oligodendrocytes [56]. Therefore, these results suggest that these cytokines maintain spared myelin by a protective mechanism and not by promotion of OPC proliferation.

GM-CSF and G-CSF also modulate the reactive astrocyte response during the first month after SCI, as seen by the reduction of GFAP levels and the CSPG neurocan [54, 55]. Another study with improvement in motor recovery by G-CSF intrathecal administration during the first day of injury also showed a reduction in the CSPG proteins neurocan and phosphocan [57]. Altogether with the previous studies, this last study suggest that G-CSF decrease the reactive gliosis because the treatment reduced TGF-β levels, a growth factor that promotes reactive gliosis; reduced vimentin levels, an astrocyte filament induced in glial scar; and presented less astrocyte proliferation [57]. Acute EPO i.p. injection also has similar results in astrocyte regulation after SCI. EPO treatment reduced lesion area and GFAP levels, while improving preservation of myelin and motor recovery at 2 wpi [58]. A following study showed possible differences with GM-CSF and G-CSF on the OPC response. Although these cytokines reduce NG2 levels, it was shown that EPO treatment increased it at 4 wpi [59].

The IL6-family of cytokines also regulates glial response. LIF i.p. administration has been shown to reduce oligodendrocyte apoptosis [60, 61], although *in vivo* LIF signalling on oligodendrocyte is not clear. On one hand, one study found that SCI induced LIFRβ expression on oligodendrocytes and that LIF treatment induced pSTAT3 and pAKT in these cells [60]. On the contrary, an alternative study did not find LIFRβ expression on oligodendrocytes and suggested a LIF positive modulation of microglia [61]. Although studies with LIF i.p. treatment have not assessed the astrocyte response in SCI, it has been shown that this treatment incremented Nestin+ cell number near the lesion site [32]. CNTF treatment, previously commented for improved motor recovery and axon regeneration, also increased the density of astrocytes [28]. Finally, gel foam administration of OSM reduced the lesion area and preserved MBP (myelin basic protein), but on the contrary to the other IL6-family cytokines, it reduced GFAP levels near the lesion site. This glial modulation was accompanied by improved serotonergic fiber outgrowth and motor recovery [15].

6.2. STAT modulation of reactive astrocytes

Contrary to motoneuron response in SCI, astrocyte response has been studied with cell-specific deletions of STAT3 and SOCS3. Deletions on Nestin or GFAP expressing cells, two genes up-regulated in reactive astrocytes, have elucidated the role of the JAK-STAT signalling pathway on reactive gliosis. Mice with Nestin:STAT3KO or GFAP:STAT3KO had an increased lesion area and decreased glial scar after 2 weeks of a contusive SCI [12, 22]. Consistent with the protective role of the glial scar, this was accompanied by increased demyelination and inflammatory response, altogether with a lack of motor recovery after injury. On the contrary, the deletion of the negative feedback in a Nestin:SOCS3KO mice had prolonged and increased pSTAT3 levels in response to SCI, resulting in reduced lesion area, early and increased glial scar surrounding this area, and improved motor recovery [12].

These *in vivo* studies demonstrated that the glial JAK-STAT signalling is necessary for secondary damage contention and further studies have elucidated the cellular mechanisms modulated by this pathway. First, it seems that JAK-STAT pathway is necessary for astrocyte survival in response to injury, as an *in vitro* study showed that GFAP:STAT3KO astrocytes had increased necrosis and protein release after a mechanical injury [62]. Besides cell survival, JAK-STAT controls gene expression associated to reactive gliosis. STAT3 controls the expression of glial filaments, as it is known that GFAP is a target gene for STAT3 [63] and in GFAP:STAT3KO mice, reduced levels of GFAP and vimentin were detected [22]. Cell morphology is also modulated by JAK-STAT pathway. In response to SCI, astrocytes near the lesion site change their cell morphology and orientation to form the glial scar. In GFAP:STAT3KO mice, astrocytes failed to change orientation and did not form the closed boundaries of the glial scar [53].

Another STAT transcription factor that controls astrocyte response is STAT5, which is activated by GM-CSF. As commented before, this cytokine reduced GFAP and CSPG levels with an increase in motor recovery [55]. An *in vitro* study with astrocytes activated with TGF-β3, which up-regulates CSPG proteins, found that GM-CSF increased pSTAT5, pAKT and pRaf levels [64]. The cytokine also reduced TGF-β signalling and CSPGs expression. GM-CSF effects were blocked by JAK and PI3K inhibitors, suggesting that STAT5 and PI3K signalling could reduce the levels of axon inhibitory proteins secreted by reactive astrocytes [64]. Following studies should clarify if STAT5 has a similar role *in vivo*.

6.3. JAK-STAT modulation of neural stem progenitor cells

Adult neural stem progenitor cells (NSPCs) can generate new astrocytes and oligodendrocytes in homeostasis and in response to injury [5, 6]. NSPCs can also generate new neurons but only in some CNS specific areas, the dentate gyrus and the subventricular zone (SVZ) [65]. The role on the JAK-STAT pathway to modulate neurogenesis and gliogenesis is not clear and probably depends on the specific context, the cytokine types and cellular phenotype. At one hand, *in vitro* studies show that the JAK-STAT pathway induces gliogenesis in opposition to neurogenic differentiation, as seen in the blocking of IL6/STAT3 axis in NSPCs [66, 67]. On the other hand, there are some *in vivo* studies that have shown a JAK-STAT role for specific cytokines in adult NSPC proliferation and neurogenesis. In the dentate gyrus, CNTF and STAT3 deficient mice had reduced NSPC proliferation and neurogenesis [68]. Using cytokine injections and deficient mice it has been also shown that IL15 and IL10 regulate NSPC proliferation in the SVZ [69, 70].

Contrary to the neurogenesis of the dentate gyrus and the SVZ, in the spinal cord there is only gliogenesis. This cell differentiation occurs in three main cell types that proliferate in response to injury: ependymal cells, astrocytes and OPCs [6]. The role of the JAK-STAT pathway on proliferation and differentiation of ependymal cells and astrocytes has not been assessed, as transgenic mice with specific cell type deletion has been done only for Nestin and GFAP promoters, which are markers for both NSPCs and mature astrocytes. On the contrary, understanding on OPCs modulation has been done *in vivo* by NG2 knockout cells [71]. In response to injury, NG2+ cells proliferate and increase in number near the lesion site. NG2 proliferation is incremented in a NG2:SOCS3KO mice. On the contrary, in the NG2:STAT3KO mice no differences in NG2 cell number and proliferation were detected [71]. This could be explained by the modulation of OPC proliferation by other STAT transcription factors or by other pathways activated by JAK proteins (**Figure 1**), which are inhibited by SOCS3. JAK-STAT modulation of NG2 cell differentiation was also assessed in this study. Although STAT3 did not regulate OPC proliferation, in the same study it was shown that NG2:STAT3KO mice had reduced differentiation to mature oligodendrocytes during the first week of injury, but not at chronic phases (1mpi) [71].

7. Role of JAK-STAT in the inflammatory response

In response to injury neutrophils, macrophages and lymphocytes infiltrate to the spinal cord [72]. There are several studies where reduction of cell infiltration improves motor recovery and tissue sparing [73, 74]. Even so, the reduction of functional recovery after SCI in mice with total ablation of infiltrated macrophages indicates that the inflammatory response is also necessary for proper recovery [75]. These differences could be explained taking into account that immune cells have different and opposite phenotypes. Microglia and macrophages, the main effectors during spinal cord inflammation, are capable of polarization that leads to either pro-inflammatory (M1 type) or anti-inflammatory cells (M2 type). While M1 macrophages participate in secondary damage as well as in axonal retraction observed after SCI, M2 macrophages are proposed to be protective and promote axonal growth [47]. Considering the role of cytokines in the regulation of the immune response, in this section we discuss studies where JAK-STAT signalling has been shown to reduce the inflammatory response or change macrophage phenotype for improvement in spinal cord functional recovery.

7.1. Anti-inflammatory cytokines

IL10 is a cytokine that has been studied in SCI for anti-inflammatory modulation and neuroprotection [46]. Endogenous IL10 expression has not been assessed in detail after SCI and it is only known that M2 infiltrated macrophages express Il10 surrounding the glial scar [75]. Using IL10 deficient mice it has been found that this cytokine is necessary for controlling the inflammatory response and apoptosis. After SCI, IL10 deficient mice have an increased expression of pro-inflammatory genes, increased levels of the pro-apoptotic proteins and decreased motor recovery [76]. Another study which replaced normal monocytes with IL10 deficient monocytes also resulted in reduced motor recovery, suggesting that this cytokine is necessary for the positive macrophage anti-inflammatory response [75]. IL10 treatments in SCI has resulted in motor recovery improvement by inflammatory and neuroprotective regulation. Acute i.p. administration of IL10 reduced lesion volume in two independent studies [77, 78]. But while one study showed that IL10 improved motor recovery and reduced TNFα expression in the injured spinal cord and in infiltrated macrophages [77], the other study did not find any functional recovery [78]. Although we previously commented other studies with motor recovery improvement by local viral over-expression of IL10 [48, 49], on those studies the inflammatory response was not assessed.

Another important anti-inflammatory cytokine is IL4, which signals by the STAT6 transcription factor. Although the neutralization of this cytokine by anti-IL4 antibody administration increased the inflammatory response, neither the IL4-neutralization treatment nor a study with STAT6 deficient mice found differences in motor recovery after SCI [79, 80]. These results indicate that Il4 signalling is not necessary for motor recovery. Further studies should test this cytokine in the promotion of the anti-inflammatory response in SCI.

In addition, there are some G-CSF studies which have shown immune modulation upon SCI. Previously commented studies for G-CSF modulation on glial cells also assessed immune response. Daily intravenous administration of G-CSF during the first 4 dpi showed that treatment not only improved motor recovery and oligodendrocyte protection, but also suppressed upregulation of the pro-inflammatory cytokines TNFα and IL1β and reduced IL1β + neutrophils infiltration [56]. Another treatment with G-CSF intrathecal injection during the first day reduced macrophage/microglia cell number and TNFα levels during the first 2 wpi

[57]. Although G-CSF is well known for neuroprotective modulation [45], only one study has elucidated a biological mechanism for G-CSF inflammatory modulation on SCI. While in this study was found an increase in microglial number at 7dpi in the G-CSF treated mice, *in vitro* analyses indicated that this cytokine induced a M2 microglial phenotype, reducing pro-inflammatory genes while inducing IL10 expression [81]. A further characterization should be done to demonstrate that G-CSF induces a M2 phenotype *in vivo*.

7.2. Pro-inflammatory cytokines

IL12 is a pro-inflammatory cytokine produced by macrophages and dendritic cells which signals via STAT4 [82]. Although it was shown that gel foam administration of IL12 regulated immune and OPC response, this treatment slightly improved motor recovery in C57BL/6 mice and did not improve function in BALB/c strain [83]. A similar result was found after SCI in STAT4 deficient mice, no improvement was found in comparison WT mice [79]. These studies suggest that IL12 signalling is not functionally important for motor recovery.

The IL6-cytokine family has shown different effects in inflammatory response after spinal cord injury. IL11 deficient mice have been assessed in SCI, with no significant differences in motor recovery or macrophage infiltration [17]. LIF treatment incremented Mac1 levels, a marker for macrophage/microglial, and IGF-1 expression on these cells [61], while gel foam administration of OSM reduced T-cell infiltration [15]. Although we previously discussed IL6 intrathecal administration for axon regeneration modulation [33, 34], IL6 is a pro-inflammatory cytokine which can be blocked to decrease inflammatory response. To avoid Il6 mediated immune response, a single i.p. administration of MR16-1, an anti-mouse IL6 receptor antibody, has been tested with positive outcomes. MR16-1 improved motor recovery after a contusive SCI [66, 84]. This treatment also reduced the lesion area, astrocyte proliferation and increased spared myelin area and neurofilament and serotonergic fibers near the lesion area [66, 85]. The mechanism underlying the MR16-1 improvement in tissue and functional recovery has been associated to microglial and infiltrated macrophage function. MR16-1 accelerated inflammatory resolution, as number of total macrophage/microglial began to decrease earlier in the treated group [85]. Further phenotypic characterization of immune cells lead to the discovery that in MR16-1 treated mice, the microglial cells had an increased phagocytic phenotype. It was also shown that macrophages had a predominant M2 phenotype and that anti-inflammatory cytokines were up-regulated while pro-inflammatory cytokines were down-regulated [84, 85].

8. Conclusion and clinical implications

Cytokine upregulation and JAK-STAT signalling activation are endogenous mechanism that are activated in response to SCI and can be used to improve motor recovery. Cell type specific and *in vitro* studies have identified the role of STATs modulation in spinal cord cells. STAT3 has been the most extensively studied STAT transcription factor in SCI, but promising results have been found in other STATs and further studies should continue to determine the roles of

STAT1 and STAT5 in SCI. Moreover, further studies with transgenic models should focus in other specific cell responses not studied up to now, like motoneuron and NSPC responses.

Several preclinical studies have shown positive outcomes for motor recovery and tissue sparing in JAK-STAT cytokine treatments (**Table 2**). Thus, modulation of the JAK-STAT signalling presents an opportunity to modulate neuron and glial response after an SCI in clinical settings. The hematopoietic cytokines have been already used in clinical studies for several pathologies, therefore are advanced in comparison with other JAK-STAT cytokines. Discussion of G-CSF and EPO treatments for SCI can be found in previous chapters [45, 86], while for GM-CSF there is one SCI clinical study finished which consisted in cytokine administration with transplant of bone marrow cells [87]. Although clinical studies have not been assessed for other cytokines in CNS trauma, there are clinical studies involving other pathologies that could be translated to SCI. The anti-inflammatory and neuroprotective mechanism of IL10 could also be assessed with a recombinant human IL10 that has been used for HIV infection and other several pathologies [46]. Emfilermin is a recombinant human LIF that has been tested, although with a lack of effectiveness, in clinical trials for embryo implantation and peripheral neuropathy [88, 89] that could also be used in SCI or other CNS diseases. Finally, tocilizumab, an anti-human IL6R, has shown positive outcomes in clinical studies for rheumatoid arthritis [90] and could be used for anti-inflammatory treatment in the spinal cord acute response.

Acknowledgements

Special thanks to Daniel Guzmán for critical reading and valuable suggestions. This work was supported by ICM (P07/011-F, P09/016-F) and FONDECYT (1141162).

Author details

Victor S. Tapia and Juan Larrain*

*Address all correspondence to: jlarrain@bio.puc.cl

Center for Aging and Regeneration, Millennium Nucleus in Regenerative Biology, Faculty of Biological Sciences, Pontifical Catholic University of Chile, Santiago, Chile

References

[1] Lee B.B., Cripps R.A., Fitzharris M., Wing P.C. The global map for traumatic spinal cord injury epidemiology: update 2011, global incidence rate. Spinal Cord. 2014;52:110–116. DOI: 10.1038/sc.2012.158

[2]   Thuret S., Moon L.D.F., Gage F.H. Therapeutic interventions after spinal cord injury. Nature Reviews Neuroscience. 2006;7(8):628–643. DOI: 10.1038/nrn1955

[3]   Cannon B. Sensation and loss. Nature. 2013;503(7475):S2–3. DOI: 10.1038/503S2a

[4]   Burda J.E., Sofroniew M.V. Reactive gliosis and the multicellular response to CNS damage and disease. Neuron. 2014;81(2):229–248. DOI: 10.1016/j.neuron.2013.12.034

[5]   Horky L., Galimi F. Fate of endogenous stem/progenitor cells following spinal cord injury. Journal of Comparative Neurology. 2006;498(4):525–538. DOI: 10.1002/cne. 21065.Fate

[6]   Barnabé-Heider F., Göritz C., Sabelström H., Takebayashi H., Pfrieger F.W., Meletis K., et al. Origin of new glial cells in intact and injured adult spinal cord. Cell Stem Cell. 2010;7(4):470–482. DOI: 10.1016/j.stem.2010.07.014

[7]   Bastien D., Lacroix S. Cytokine pathways regulating glial and leukocyte function after spinal cord and peripheral nerve injury. Experimental Neurology. 2014;258:62–77. DOI: 10.1016/j.expneurol.2014.04.006

[8]   Kundi S., Bicknell R., Ahmed Z. The role of angiogenic and wound-healing factors after spinal cord injury in mammals. Neuroscience Research. 2013;76:1–9. DOI: 10.1016/ j.neures.2013.03.013

[9]   Murray P. The JAK-STAT signaling pathway: input and output integration. The Journal of Immunology. 2007;178:2623–2629. DOI: 10.4049/jimmunol.178.5.2623

[10] Rawlings J.S., Rosler K.M., Harrison D. The JAK/STAT signaling pathway. Journal of Cell Science. 2004;117:1281–1283. DOI: 10.1242/jcs.00963

[11] Smith P., Sun F., Park K., Cai B., Wang C. SOCS3 deletion promotes optic nerve regeneration in vivo. Neuron. 2009;64(5):617–623. DOI: 10.1016/j.neuron. 2009.11.021.SOCS3

[12] Okada S., Nakamura M., Katoh H., Miyao T., Shimazaki T., Ishii K., et al. Conditional ablation of Stat3 or Socs3 discloses a dual role for reactive astrocytes after spinal cord injury. Nature Medicine. 2006;12(7):829–834. DOI: 10.1038/nm1425

[13] Jin D., Liu Y., Sun F., Wang X., Liu X., He Z. Restoration of skilled locomotion by sprouting corticospinal axons induced by co-deletion of PTEN and SOCS3. Nature Communications. 2015;6:8074. DOI: 10.1038/ncomms9074

[14] Pineau I., Lacroix S. Proinflammatory cytokine synthesis in the injured mouse spinal cord: multiphasic expression pattern and identification of the cell types involved. Journal of Comparative Neurology. 2007;500(2):267–285. DOI: 10.1002/cne

[15] Slaets H., Nelissen S., Janssens K., Vidal P.M., Lemmens E., Stinissen P., et al. Oncostatin M reduces lesion size and promotes functional recovery and neurite outgrowth after spinal cord injury. Molecular Neurobiology. 2014;50(3):1142–1151. DOI: 10.1007/ s12035-014-8795-5

[16] Yamauchi K., Osuka K., Takayasu M., Usuda N., Nakazawa A., Nakahara N., et al. Activation of JAK/STAT signalling in neurons following spinal cord injury in mice. Journal of Neurochemistry. 2006;96(4):1060–1070. DOI: 10.1111/j. 1471-4159.2005.03559.x

[17] Cho N., Nguyen D.H., Satkunendrarajah K., Branch D.R., Fehlings M.G. Evaluating the role of IL-11, a novel cytokine in the IL-6 family, in a mouse model of spinal cord injury. Journal of Neuroinflammation. 2012;9:134. DOI: 10.1186/1742-2094-9-134

[18] Tripathi R.B., McTigue D.M. Chronically increased ciliary neurotrophic factor and fibroblast growth factor-2 expression after spinal contusion in rats. Journal of Comparative Neurology. 2008;510(2):129–144. DOI: 10.1002/cne.21787

[19] Hesp Z.C., Goldstein E.Z., Goldstein E., Miranda C.J., Kaspar B.K., et al. Chronic oligodendrogenesis and remyelination after spinal cord injury in mice and rats. Journal of Neuroscience. 2015;35(3):1274–1290. DOI: 10.1523/JNEUROSCI.2568-14.2015

[20] Osuka K., Watanabe Y., Usuda N., Atsuzawa K., Yasuda M., Aoshima C., et al. Activation of STAT1 in neurons following spinal cord injury in mice. Neurochemical Research. 2011;36(12):2236–2243. DOI: 10.1007/s11064-011-0547-6

[21] Park K., Lin C., Lee Y. Expression of suppressor of cytokine signaling-3 (SOCS3) and its role in neuronal death after complete spinal cord injury. Experimental Neurology. 2014;0:65–75. DOI: 10.1016/j.expneurol.2014.06.013

[22] Herrmann J.E., Imura T., Song B., Qi J., Ao Y., Thu K., et al. STAT3 is a critical regulator of astrogliosis and scar formation after spinal cord injury. Journal of Neuroscience. 2009;28(28):7231–7243. DOI: 10.1523/JNEUROSCI.1709-08.2008.

[23] Tuszynski M.H., Steward O. Concepts and methods for the study of axonal regeneration in the CNS. Neuron. 2012;74(5):777–791. DOI: 10.1016/j.neuron.2012.05.006

[24] Bareyre F.M., Kerschensteiner M., Raineteau O., Mettenleiter T.C., Weinmann O., Schwab M.E. The injured spinal cord spontaneously forms a new intraspinal circuit in adult rats. Nature Neuroscience. 2004;7(3):269–277. DOI: 10.1038/nn1195

[25] Weidner N., Ner A. Spontaneous corticospinal axonal plasticity and functional recovery after adult central nervous system injury. Proceedings of the National Academy of Sciences of the United States of America. 2001;98(6):3513–3518. DOI: 10.1073/pnas.051626798

[26] Bareyre F.M., Garzorz N., Lang C., Misgeld T., Büning H., Kerschensteiner M. In vivo imaging reveals a phase-specific role of STAT3 during central and peripheral nervous system axon regeneration. Proceedings of the National Academy of Sciences of the United States of America. 2011;108(15):6282–62787. DOI: 10.1073/pnas.1015239108

[27] Lang C., Bradley P.M., Jacobi A., Kerschensteiner M., Bareyre F.M. STAT3 promotes corticospinal remodelling and functional recovery after spinal cord injury. EMBO Reports. 2013;14(10):931–937. DOI: 10.1038/embor.2013.117

[28] Ye J., Cao L., Cui R., Huang A., Yan Z., Lu C., et al. The effects of ciliary neurotrophic factor on neurological function and glial activity following contusive spinal cord injury in the rats. Brain Research. 2004;997(1):30–39. DOI: 10.1016/j.brainres.2003.10.036

[29] Wang N., Zhang S., Zhang F., Yang Z.Y., Li X.G. Sodium hyaluronate-CNTF gelatinous particles promote axonal growth, neurogenesis and functional recovery after spinal cord injury. Spinal Cord. 2014;52(7):517–523. DOI: 10.1038/sc.2014.54

[30] Pitzer C., Klussmann S., Krüger C., Letellier E., Plaas C., Dittgen T., et al. The hematopoietic factor granulocyte-colony stimulating factor improves outcome in experimental spinal cord injury. Journal of Neurochemistry. 210;113(4):930–942. DOI: 10.1111/j.1471-4159.2010.06659.x

[31] Pan W., Cain C., Yu Y., Kastin A.J. Receptor-mediated transport of LIF across blood-spinal cord barrier is upregulated after spinal cord injury. Journal of Neuroimmunology. 2006;174:119–125. DOI: 10.1016/j.jneuroim.2006.02.006

[32] Li Y., Zang D. The neuron regrowth is associated with the proliferation of neural precursor cells after leukemia inhibitory factor administration following spinal cord injury in mice. PloS One. 2014;9(12):e116031. DOI: 10.1371/journal.pone.0116031

[33] Yang P., Wen H., Ou S., Cui J., Fan D. IL-6 promotes regeneration and functional recovery after cortical spinal tract injury by reactivating intrinsic growth program of neurons and enhancing synapse formation. Experimental Neurology. 2012;236:19–27. DOI: 10.1016/j.expneurol.2012.03.019

[34] Yang P., Qin Y., Bian C., Zhao Y., Zhang W. Intrathecal delivery of IL-6 reactivates the intrinsic growth capacity of pyramidal cells in the sensorimotor cortex after spinal cord injury. PloS One. 2015;10(5):e0127772. DOI: 10.1371/journal.pone.0127772

[35] Zhang Y., Xiong Y., Mahmood A., Meng Y., Liu Z. Sprouting of corticospinal tract axons from the contralateral hemisphere into the denervated side of the spinal cord is associated with functional recovery in adult rat. Brain Research. 2010;1353:249–257. DOI: 10.1016/j.brainres.2010.07.046

[36] Stephanou A., Brar B. Opposing actions of STAT-1 and STAT-3 on the Bcl-2 and Bcl-x promoters. Cell Death and Differentiation. 2000;7(3):329–330.

[37] Silva M., Benito A., Sanz C., Prosper F. Erythropoietin can induce the expression of bcl-xLthrough stat5 in erythropoietin-dependent progenitor cell lines. Journal of Biological Chemistry. 1999;274(32):22165–22169.

[38] Zhou Z., Peng X., Insolera R. Interleukin-10 provides direct trophic support to neurons. Journal of Neurochemistry. 2009;110(5):1617–1627. DOI: 10.1111/j.1471-4159.2009.06263.x.

[39] Park K.W., Nozell S.E., Benveniste E.N. Protective role of STAT3 in NMDA and glutamate-induced neuronal death: negative regulatory effect of SOCS3. PloS One. 1012;7(11):e50874. DOI: 10.1371/journal.pone.0050874

[40] Nishio Y., Koda M., Kamada T. Granulocyte colony-stimulating factor attenuates neuronal death and promotes functional recovery after spinal cord injury in mice. Journal of Neuropathology and Experimental Neurology. 2997;66(8):724–731.

[41] Takagi Y., Harada J., Chiarugi A., Moskowitz M. STAT1 is activated in neurons after ischemia and contributes to ischemic brain injury. Journal of Cerebral Blood Flow and Metabolism. 2002;22(11):1311–1318. DOI: 10.1097/01.WCB.0000034148.72481.F4

[42] Loddick S., Turnbull A., Rothwell N. Cerebral interleukin-6 is neuroprotective during permanent focal cerebral ischemia in the rat. Journal of Cerebral Blood Flow and Metabolis. 1998;18:176–17.

[43] Yamashita T., Sawamoto K., Suzuki S., Suzuki N., Adachi K., Kawase T., et al. Blockade of interleukin-6 signaling aggravates ischemic cerebral damage in mice: possible involvement of Stat3 activation in the protection of neurons. Journal of Neurochemistry. 2005;94(2):459–68. DOI: 10.1111/j.1471-4159.2005.03227.x

[44] Schweizer U., Gunnersen J., Karch C., Wiese S., Holtmann B., Takeda K., et al. Conditional gene ablation of Stat3 reveals differential signaling requirements for survival of motoneurons during development and after nerve injury in the adult. Journal of Cell Biology. 2002;156(2):287–97. DOI: 10.1083/jcb.200107009

[45] Wallner S., Peters S., Pitzer C., Resch H., Bogdahn U., Schneider A. The granulocyte-colony stimulating factor has a dual role in neuronal and vascular plasticity. Frontiers in Cell and Developmental Biology. 2015;3:48. DOI: 10.3389/fcell.2015.00048

[46] Thompson C.D., Zurko J.C., Hanna B.F., Hellenbrand D.J., Hanna A. The therapeutic role of interleukin-10 after spinal cord injury. Journal of Neurotrauma. 2013;30:1311–1324. DOI: 10.1089/neu.2012.2651

[47] David S., Kroner A. Repertoire of microglial and macrophage responses after spinal cord injury. Nature Reviews Neuroscience. 2011;12(7):388–399. DOI: 10.1038/nrn3053

[48] Zhou Z., Peng X., Insolera R., Fink D., Mata M. IL-10 promotes neuronal survival following spinal cord injury. Experimental Neurology. 2009;220(1):183–190. DOI: 10.1016/j.expneurol.2009.08.018

[49] Jackson C., Messinger J., Peduzzi J.D., Ansardi D.C., Morrow C.D. Enhanced functional recovery from spinal cord injury following intrathecal or intramuscular administration of poliovirus replicons encoding IL-10. Virology. 2005;336(2):173–183. DOI: 10.1016/j.virol.2005.03.025

[50] Park K.W., Lin C.Y., Li K., Lee Y.S. Effects of reducing suppressors of cytokine signaling-3 (SOCS3) expression on dendritic outgrowth and demyelination after spinal cord injury. PloS One. 2015;10(9):e0138301. DOI: 10.1371/journal.pone.0138301

[51] Yiu G., He Z. Glial inhibition of CNS axon regeneration. Nature Reviews Neuroscience. 2006;7(8):617–627. DOI: 10.1038/nrn1956.

[52] Faulkner J.R., Herrmann J.E., Woo M.J., Tansey K.E., Doan N.B., Sofroniew M.V. Reactive astrocytes protect tissue and preserve function after spinal cord injury. Journal of Neuroscience. 2004;24(9):2143–2155. DOI: 10.1523/JNEUROSCI.3547-03.2004

[53] Wanner I.B., Anderson M., Song B., Levine J., Fernandez A., Gray-Thompson Z., et al. Glial scar borders are formed by newly proliferated, elongated astrocytes that interact to corral inflammatory and fibrotic cells via STAT3-dependent mechanisms after spinal cord injury. Journal of Neuroscience. 2013;33(31):12870–12886. DOI: 10.1523/JNEUROSCI.2121-13.2013

[54] Huang X., Kim J.M., Kong T.H., Park S.R., Ha Y., Kim M.H., et al. GM-CSF inhibits glial scar formation and shows long-term protective effect after spinal cord injury. Journal of the Neurological Science. 2009;277:87–97. DOI: 10.1016/j.jns.2008.10.02

[55] Chung J., Kim M., Yoon Y., Kim K. Effects of granulocyte colony–stimulating factor and granulocyte-macrophage colony–stimulating factor on glial scar formation after spinal cord injury in rats. Journal of Neurosurgery: Spine. 2014;21(6):966–973. DOI: 10.3171/2014.8.SPINE131090

[56] Kadota R., Koda M., Kawabe J., Hashimoto M., Nishio Y., Mannoji C., et al. Granulocyte colony-stimulating factor (G–CSF) protects oligodendrocyte and promotes hindlimb functional recovery after spinal cord injury in rats. PloS One. 2012;7(11):e50391. DOI: 10.1371/journal.pone.0050391

[57] Chen W.F., Chen C.H., Chen N.F., Sung C.S., Wen Z.H. Neuroprotective effects of direct intrathecal administration of granulocyte colony-stimulating factor in rats with spinal cord injury. CNS Neuroscience & Therapeutics. 2015;21(9):698–707. DOI: 10.1111/cns.12429

[58] Gorio A., Madaschi L. Methylprednisolone neutralizes the beneficial effects of erythropoietin in experimental spinal cord injury. Proceedings of the National Academy of Sciences of the United States of America. 2005;102(45):16379–16384. DOI: 10.1073/pnas.0508479102

[59] Vitellaro-Zuccarello L., Mazzetti S., Madaschi L., Bosisio P., Gorio A., De Biasi S. Erythropoietin-mediated preservation of the white matter in rat spinal cord injury. Neuroscience. 2007;144(3):865–877. DOI: 10.1016/j.neuroscience.2006.10.023

[60] Azari M., Profyris C. Leukemia inhibitory factor arrests oligodendrocyte death and demyelination in spinal cord injury. Journal of Neuropathology and Experimental Neurology. 2006;65(6):914–929. DOI: 10.1097/01.jnen.0000235855.77716.25

[61] Kerr B.J., Patterson P.H. Leukemia inhibitory factor promotes oligodendrocyte survival after spinal cord injury. Glia. 2005;51:73–79. DOI: 10.1002/glia.20177

[62] Levine J., Kwon E., Paez P., Yan W., Czerwieniec G., Loo J., et al. Traumatically injured astrocytes release a proteomic signature modulated by STAT3-dependent cell survival. Glia. 2015; 64(5):668-694. DOI: 10.1002/glia.22953

[63] Takizawa T., Nakashima K., Namihira M. DNA methylation is a critical cell-intrinsic determinant of astrocyte differentiation in the fetal brain. Developmental Cell. 2001;1(6):749–758. DOI: 10.1016/S1534-5807(01)00101-0

[64] Choi J., Park S., Kim K., Park S. GM-CSF reduces expression of chondroitin sulfate proteoglycan (CSPG) core proteins in TGF-β-treated primary astrocytes. BMB Reports. 2014;47(12):679–684. DOI: 10.5483/BMBRep.2014.47.12.018

[65] Alvarez-Buylla A., Seri B., Doetsch F. Identification of neural stem cells in the adult vertebrate brain. Brain Research Bulletin. 2002;57(6):751–758. DOI: 10.1016/S0361-9230(01)00770-5

[66] Okada S., Nakamura M., Mikami Y., Shimazaki T., Mihara M., Ohsugi Y., et al. Blockade of interleukin-6 receptor suppresses reactive astrogliosis and ameliorates functional recovery in experimental spinal cord injury. Journal of Neuroscience Research. 2004;76(2):265–276. DOI: 10.1002/jnr.20044

[67] Gu F., Hata R., Ma Y.J., Tanaka J., Mitsuda N., Kumon Y., et al. Suppression of Stat3 promotes neurogenesis in cultured neural stem cells. Journal of Neuroscience Research. 2005;81(2):163–171. DOI: 10.1002/jnr.20561

[68] Müller S., Chakrapani B.P.S., Schwegler H., Hofmann H.D., Kirsch M. Neurogenesis in the dentate gyrus depends on ciliary neurotrophic factor and signal transducer and activator of transcription 3 signaling. Stem Cells. 2009;27(2):431–441. DOI: 10.1634/stemcells.2008-0234

[69] Gómez-Nicola D., Valle-Argos B., Pallas-Bazarra N., Nieto-Sampedro M. Interleukin-15 regulates proliferation and self-renewal of adult neural stem cells. Molecular Biology of the Cell. 2011;22:1960–1970. DOI: 10.1091/mbc.E11-01-0053

[70] Pereira L., Font-Nieves M., Van den Haute C., Baekelandt V., Planas A.M., Pozas E. IL-10 regulates adult neurogenesis by modulating ERK and STAT3 activity. Frontiers in Cellular Neuroscience. 2015;9:57. DOI: 10.3389/fncel.2015.00057

[71] Hackett A.R., Lee D.H., Dawood A., Rodriguez M., Funk L., Tsoulfas P., et al. STAT3 and SOCS3 regulate NG2 cell proliferation and differentiation after contusive spinal cord injury. Neurobiology of Disease. 2016;89:10–22. DOI: 10.1016/j.nbd.2016.01.017

[72] Prüss H., Kopp M., Brommer B., Gatzemeier N., Laginha I., Dirnagl U., et al. Non-resolving aspects of acute inflammation after spinal cord injury (SCI): indices and resolution plateau. Brain Pathology. 2011;21(6):652–660. DOI: 10.1111/j.1750-3639.2011.00488.x

[73] Popovich P.G., Guan Z., Wei P., Huitinga I., van Rooijen N., Stokes B.T. Depletion of hematogenous macrophages promotes partial hindlimb recovery and neuroanatomical repair after experimental spinal cord injury. Experimental Neurology. 1999;158:351–365. DOI: 10.1006/exnr.1999.7118

[74] Saville L.R., Pospisil C.H., Mawhinney L.A., Bao F., Simedrea F.C., Peters A.A., et al. A monoclonal antibody to CD11d reduces the inflammatory infiltrate into the injured

spinal cord: A potential neuroprotective treatment. Journal of Neuroimmunology. 2004;156:42–57. DOI: 10.1016/j.jneuroim.2004.07.002

[75] Shechter R., London A., Varol C., Raposo C., Cusimano M., Yovel G., et al. Infiltrating blood-derived macrophages are vital cells playing an anti-inflammatory role in recovery from spinal cord injury in mice. PLoS Medicine. 2009;6(7):e1000113. DOI: 10.1371/journal.pmed.1000113

[76] Genovese T., Esposito E., Mazzon E., Di Paola R., Caminiti R., Bramanti P., et al. Absence of endogenous interleukin-10 enhances secondary inflammatory process after spinal cord compression injury in mice. Journal of Neurochemistry. 2009;108(6):1360–1372. DOI: 10.1111/j.1471-4159.2009.05899.x

[77] Bethea J.R., Nagashima H., Acosta M.C., Briceno C., Gomez F., Marcillo A.E., et al. Systemically administered interleukin-10 reduces tumor necrosis factor-alpha production and significantly improves functional recovery following traumatic spinal cord. Journal of Neurotrauma. 1999;16(10):851–863. DOI: 10.1089/neu.1999.16.851

[78] Takami T., Oudega M., Bethea J.R., Wood P.M., Kleitman N., Bunge M.B. Methylprednisolone and interleukin-10 reduce gray matter damage in the contused Fischer rat thoracic spinal cord but do not improve functional outcome. Journal of Neurotrauma. 2002;19(5):653–666. DOI: 10.1089/089771502753754118

[79] Fraidakis M., Kiyotani T., Pernold K. Recovery from spinal cord injury in tumor necrosis factor-alpha, signal transducers and activators of transcription 4 and signal transducers and activators of transcription 6 null mice. Neuroimmunology. 2007;18(2): 185–189.

[80] Lee S.I., Jeong S.R., Kang Y.M., Han D.H., Jin B.K., Namgung U., et al. Endogenous expression of interleukin-4 regulates macrophage activation and confines cavity formation after traumatic spinal cord injury. Journal of Neuroscience Research. 2010;88:2409–2419. DOI: 10.1002/jnr.22411

[81] Guo Y., Zhang H., Yang J., Liu S., Bing L., Gao J., et al. Granulocyte colony-stimulating factor improves alternative activation of microglia under microenvironment of spinal cord injury. Neuroscience. 2013;238:1–10. DOI: 10.1016/j.neuroscience. 2013.01.047

[82] Vignali D., Kuchroo V.K. IL-12 family cytokines: immunological playmakers. Nature Immunology. 2012;13(8):722–728. DOI: 10.1038/ni.2366

[83] Yaguchi M., Ohta S., Toyama Y., Kawakami Y., Toda M. Functional recovery after spinal cord injury in mice through activation of microglia and dendritic cells after IL-12 administration. Journal of Neuroscience Research. 2008;86(9):1972–1980. DOI: 10.1002/ jnr.21658

[84] Guerrero A.R., Uchida K., Nakajima H., Watanabe S., Nakamura M., Johnson W.E., et al. Blockade of interleukin-6 signaling inhibits the classic pathway and promotes an

alternative pathway of macrophage activation after spinal cord injury in mice. Journal of Neuroinflammation. 2012;9:40. DOI: 10.1186/1742-2094-9-40

[85] Mukaino M., Nakamura M., Yamada O., Okada S., Morikawa S., Renault-Mihara F., et al. Anti-IL-6-receptor antibody promotes repair of spinal cord injury by inducing microglia-dominant inflammation. Experimental Neurology. 2010;224:403–414. DOI: 10.1016/j.expneurol.2010.04.020

[86] Carelli S., Marfia G., Di Giulio A.M., Ghilardi G., Gorio A. Erythropoietin: recent developments in the treatment of spinal cord injury. Neurology Research International. 2011;2011:453179. DOI: 10.1155/2011/453179

[87] Yoon S.H., Shim Y.S., Park Y.H., Chung J.K., Nam J.H., Kim M.O., et al. Complete spinal cord injury treatment using autologous bone marrow cell transplantation and bone marrow stimulation with granulocyte macrophage-colony stimulating factor: Phase I/II clinical trial. Stem Cells. 2007;25(8):2066–2073. DOI: 10.1634/stemcells.2006-0807

[88] Davis I.D., Kiers L., MacGregor L., Quinn M., Arezzo J., Green M., et al. A randomized, double-blinded, placebo-controlled phase II trial of recombinant human leukemia inhibitory factor (rhuLIF, emfilermin, AM424) to prevent chemotherapy-induced peripheral neuropathy. Clinical Cancer Research. 2005;11:1890–1898. DOI: 10.1158/1078-0432.CCR-04-1655

[89] Brinsden P.R., Alam V., de Moustier B., Engrand P. Recombinant human leukemia inhibitory factor does not improve implantation and pregnancy outcomes after assisted reproductive techniques in women with recurrent unexplained implantation failure. Fertility and Sterility. 2009;91:1445–1447. DOI: 10.1016/j.fertnstert.2008.06.047

[90] Hashizume M., Tan S.L., Takano J., Ohsawa K., Hasada I., Hanasaki A., et al. Tocilizumab, a humanized anti-IL-6R antibody, as an emerging therapeutic option for rheumatoid arthritis: molecular and cellular mechanistic insights. International Reviews of Immunology. 2015;34(3):265–279. DOI: 10.3109/08830185.2014.938325

5

Understanding Molecular Pathology along Injured Spinal Cord Axis: Moving Frontiers toward Effective Neuroprotection and Regeneration

Dasa Cizkova, Adriana-Natalia Murgoci,
Lenka Kresakova, Katarina Vdoviakova, Milan Cizek,
Tomas Smolek, Veronika Cubinkova, Jusal Quanico,
Isabelle Fournier and Michel Salzet

Abstract

Spinal cord injury (SCI) is a severe, often life threatening, traumatic condition leading to serious neurological dysfunctions. The pathological hallmarks of SCI include inflammation, reactive gliosis, axonal demyelination, neuronal death, and cyst formation. Although much has been learned about the progression of SCI pathology affecting a large number of biochemical cascades and reactions, the roles of proteins involved in these processes are not well understood. Advances in proteomic technologies have made it possible to examine the spinal cord proteome from healthy and experimental animals and disclose a detailed overview on the spatial and temporal regionalization of these secondary processes. Data clearly demonstrated that neurotrophic molecules dominated in the segment above the central lesion, while the proteins associated with necrotic/apoptotic pathways abound the segment below the lesion. This knowledge is extremely important in finding optimal targets and pathways on which complementary neuroprotective and neuroregenerative approaches should be focused on. In terms of neuroprotection, several active substances and cell-based therapy together with biomaterials releasing bioactive substances showed partial improvement of spinal cord injury. However, one of the major challenges is to select specific therapies that can be combined safely and in the appropriate order to provide the maximum value of each individual treatment.

Keywords: spinal cord injury, secondary processes, proteome, biomaterials

1. Introduction

Intensive lifestyle brought about by the modern age of the twenty-first century often brings risks of trauma to the CNS. Both trauma of brain and spinal cord are considered not only as life-threatening conditions, but also as substantial, social, and economic problems that affect mainly the young population. The increased incidence of trauma may be related to popular sports such as ice hockey, American football, rugby, horse riding, and diving, but the most common causes include traffic accidents [1]. Spinal cord trauma accounts for 70% of the total number of CNS injuries.

Many spinal cord (SCI) patients remain permanently paralyzed with complete or partial loss of neurological functions below the site of injury [2]. The most common is paralysis of the body, usually affecting both lower limbs. At the same time, complications may arise when loss of sensitivity, urinary tract control, or the development of spasticity occur in the affected area [3]. Statistics shows that victims are twice as often men as women, with the highest occurrence of cases between the 19 and 40 years of age [4]. Care for patients with injured spinal cord is demanding and often requires lifelong financial costs [4].

The neurological outcomes depend on the range of damaged neuronal populations at the injury site, the level of disconnection of ascending and descending neuronal pathways, the secondary damage (edema, inflammation, and ischemia), and the age-dependent activation of regenerative processes (endogenous production of trophic factors and revascularization). Thus, patients with incomplete injury who retain some sensory or motor function below the lesion, undergo an extensive rehabilitation program to have a better chance of recovering some function. On the contrary, severe spinal cord injury causes a life-lasting disability for which currently no effective therapy is available. Another important factor is age; statistics shows that younger patients have better prognosis of recovery.

Therefore, the main objective of biomedical research is the development of new therapeutic procedures that would contribute to a more effective functional outcome and improvement of the quality of life.

In this chapter, we would like to highlight pathological consequences that could be evaluated by temporal and spatial proteomic analyses, leading to discrimination of the proteome within the entire spinal cord after acute injury. These data will be correlated with delivery of individual neuroprotective and combinatory neuroregenerative strategies for SCI treatment.

2. Pathology

Spinal cord trauma triggers a pathophysiological complex of cellular and molecular reactions leading to edema, hemorrhage, free radical formation, glutamate excitotoxicity, ischemia, macrophage phagocytic activation, glial scar formation, and apoptotic changes in the injured tissue [5]. These processes take place within a few minutes to weeks and years after the injury.

During this time, under the influence of secondary events, small primary damage will spread to the surrounding healthy area within the craniocaudal axis, causing partial or complete loss of physiological functions below the site of injury.

One of the key events of secondary processes is inflammation characterized by fluid accumulation (edema) and the recruitment of immune cells (neutrophils, T-cells, macrophages, and monocytes) [6]. In fact, spinal cord microglial cells normally function as a kind of reactive immune cells that begin to respond to signals after pathological stimuli (injury, infection, or tumors) [7] and are activated at the lesion epicenter [8]. It has been suggested that microglia/macrophages can be polarized into M1-neurotoxic or M2-neuroprotective states and produce a variety of cytokines, chemokines, and neurotrophic factors. However, the mechanisms regulating microglial polarity remain unclear [9].

In addition, not only stimulated microglia/macrophages but also astrocytes, meningeal cells, and fibroblasts together with the increased production of inhibitory chondroitin sulfate proteoglycans (CSPGs) are involved in the spinal cord pathogenesis [10]. Macrophages can alter their phenotypes and functions according to changes in the spinal cord microenvironment during subacute and chronic phases. Thus, SCI triggers an excessive inflammatory response mediated by the invasion of M1/M2 macrophages into and around the central lesion at subacute phase, but not at chronic phase when the formation of glial scar occurs.

2.1. Neuroinflammation

In the CNS, immune cells acquire diverse phenotypes depending on the pathophysiology of the microenvironment.

The inflammatory environment of injured spinal cord contains pro-inflammatory cytokines such as tumor necrosis factor α (TNFα), interleukins IL-1 and IL -6. Anti-inflammatory molecules, like transforming growth factor β1 (TGFβ) and IL-10, are released as well. Immune response in the CNS is mediated by resident microglia and astrocytes, which are innate immune cells without direct counterparts in the periphery.

Among glial cells, microglia are firstly activated and are able to play a bifunctional role. They secrete toxic factors and contribute to tissue damage, but at the same time also release neuroprotective and neurotrophic molecules to allow tissue repair [11]. Interestingly, microglia and astrocytes are able to cross-talk with CNS-infiltrating immune cells, such as neutrophils, T cells, and other components of the innate immune system, as well as with neurons.

Neutrophils are considered as the first inflammatory cells to arrive at the site of injury with a peak at 24 h after injury [12]. They are rapidly mobilized from the bone marrow in response to signals from pro-inflammatory CXC (CXCL8) family chemokines, IL- and cytokine-induced neutrophil chemoattractant 1 (CINC-1) to mediate pleiotropic functions in the immune-inflammatory response [13]. Neutrophils adhere to post-capillary venules 6–12 h post SCI and afterwards they migrate into the lesion site to phagocytose debris [14]. Neutrophils generate their own cytokines after stimulation by pro-inflammatory mediators and produce proteases via the NF-kB translocation pathway. Phagocytic activity can induce NF-kB activation [15, 16], and other mediators such as matrix metalloproteases (MMPs), and cytokines TNFα, IL-1, IL-8, and TGF-β [17].

Microglia are a unique myeloid cell population, derived from the yolk sac during a narrow time window during development (before vascularization or definitive hematopoiesis) in the embryo. Microglia cells, present in the CNS parenchyma, are sustained by the proliferation of resident progenitors, independently of blood cells.

Their response following pathological stimuli is characterized by an accumulation at the lesion site and the release of various bioactive molecules. Two categories of molecules are released, some are cytotoxic or pro-inflammatory, and others may aid survival and regeneration. Resident monocytes are the first cell types to respond after injury within 1–2 h, which starts the initial acute inflammatory response accompanied by an expression of TNFα and IL-1 (M1 phenotype). This leads to the recruitment of other immune cells. M1 macrophages promote phagocytosis. Eight hours after injury, the production of pro-inflammatory cytokines is terminated, thus promoting the differentiation of macrophages into an anti-inflammatory M2 phenotype with the expression of arginase 1 and a mannose receptor (CD206). M2 macrophages promote angiogenesis and matrix remodeling, while suppressing destructive immunity [18]. The ratio M1/M2 varies in terms of the microenvironment.

These findings correlate with accumulating evidence pointing to a chronological time line expression of different degeneration- and regeneration-associated genes that are involved in the pathogenesis and endogenous repair or plasticity during days to months following SCI.

2.2. Neuro-glial interactions

Microglia activation may be beneficial, deleterious or neutral [8, 9]. Neurons express cell surface glycoproteins (CD22, CD47, CD200, and NCAM) to prevent microglia activation [10, 19]. A relationship between the nervous and immune system has been studied this past decade. Indeed, glial cells (microglia and astrocytes) not only perform supportive and nutritive roles for neurons, but also serve to defend the CNS. On the other hand, excessive and prolonged glial cell activation may result in more severe and chronic neuronal damage, leading to neuroinflammation and neurodegeneration [11, 13].

Neurons are able to control microglia with two types of signals: "On" or "Off" [20]. Off signals (TGF-β, CD22, CX3CL1, neurotransmitters, and CD20) are found in healthy conditions to maintain homeostasis and also restrict microglial activities under inflammatory conditions to prevent damage to healthy tissue. Conversely, "On" signals [CCL21, CXCL10, and MMP3 (from apoptotic neurons)] are produced by damaged and impaired neurons to activate microglia (pro- or anti-inflammatory) [21].

2.3. Glial scar

Glial scar is the accompanying pathological phenomenon of various CNS injuries. The site of injury is infiltrated by macrophages from the bloodstream, fibroblasts, astrocytes, microglia, and oligodendrocytes [8]. Later, precursors of oligodendrocytes and meningeal cells are activated.

Activated astrocytes proliferate and, together with other glial cells, produce a glial scar that encloses the lesion site and prevents the diffusion of ions, neurotransmitters, and other metabolites from damaged tissue into surrounding healthy tissue [22]. This protects undamaged tissue from inflammation and demyelinization, while at the same time, it also prevents regeneration of nerve fibers, which is a serious problem for the treatment of spinal cord injuries. Activated astrocytes reveal thicker projections that intersect with each other and are connected by tight joints. Astrogliosis is accompanied by increased expression of glial fibrillary acidic protein (GFAP), vimentin, and markers for neural precursor cells (Nestin) [23]. In reactive astrocytes, increased synthesis of extracellular matrix protein CSPGs has been reported, which are inhibitory to axon growth itself [23]. Similarly, oligodendroglia, together with meningeal cells migrating into the lesion, form a significant barrier for axonal growth by producing inhibitory molecules (NOGO) and other proteoglycans [24].

2.4. Inhibitory molecules

NOGO inhibitory protein [25, 26], myelin glycoprotein oligodendrocyte (OMGP) [27], myelin-associated glycoprotein (MAG) [28] together with secondary inhibitors, including the large group of chondroitin sulfate proteoglycans (CSPGs), are among the major inhibitory molecules that block axonal regeneration [24, 29]. While blocking the penetration of axons, they contribute to the formation of so-called blind clusters, unable to form functional connections with terminal neurons. These pathological formations often cause painful irritable syndrome [30].

Inhibitory CSPGs are synthesized by neurons and glial cells. They play an important role in the physiological development of the CNS, such as cell migration, maturation, differentiation, survival, and tissue homeostasis, but in the case of disruption of tissue homeostasis, increase their expression and consequently inhibit regeneration [31]. These molecules interact extensively with extracellular matrix components [32], for example, with laminin, fibronectin, tenascin, and collagen [33]. Additionally, they bind to growth factors, midkine, pleiotrophin, fibroblast growth factor [34], or inhibitory growth factors such as semaphorins [19] and contribute to the formation of a glial scar that inhibits regeneration of axons [35]. NG2 glycoprotein, which belongs to the most important inhibitors of the CSPGs group, is produced by oligodendrocytes precursor, meningeal cells and macrophages [36]. Accumulation of NG2 was seen at the site of injury, where it blocks regeneration of the axons [31]. Co-expression of NG2 and PDGF-α receptors in the same population of CNS cells confirmed its specific expression in oligodendrocyte precursors [37]. NG2-positive oligodendrocyte precursor cells are often the first cells to respond to injury. Unlike microglia, reactive oligodendrocyte changes are local and occur only in the immediate vicinity of the injury. Previous experiments confirm the initiation of spontaneous regeneration in SCI, as reflected by the incidence of GAP-43-positive axons. They were found in the segments above the lesion at first week [38]. In the central lesion, which forms a mechanical and chemical barrier, the inhibitory proteoglycan NG2 was significantly enhanced [39]. Immunohistochemical analyses using specific NG2/GAP-43 antibody confirmed that increased accumulation of NG2-positive cells at the central injury creates a barrier for successful diffusion and further ingrowth of GAP-43-labeled axonal fibers at acute phase [38]. Sequential administration of ChABC enzyme caused degradation of NG2 glycoprotein, which modified the extracellular matrix and created a tolerant environment for longer term recovery (2–3 weeks).

2.5. Neuropathological consequences based on proteomic analyses

Based on the recent analyses of SCI pathological processes, it seems that complex changes in gene and protein expression as well as in cellular interactions are taking place not only at the central lesion but also in adjacent segments. However, the exact mechanisms by which proteins involved during inflammation, recruitment and microglia activation, glial scaring, remyelination, or axonal growth function remain to be further explored [5, 10, 21, 35]. Therefore, understanding of the molecular cross-talk occurring between cells at the lesion site and in the adjacent segments needs to be further investigated [21]. In particular, studies that are able to take into account both spatial and temporal data may identify interesting molecular targets [40]. Such an investigation could be performed by a **proteomics approach**, which can be connected to cellular and physiological studies as well as to a global regeneration-activated gene (RAG) investigation. Mass spectrometry (MS) plays a central role among proteomics approaches. Several developments allow fast identification of lower abundance proteins such as cytokines and chemokines [41]. Furthermore, MS is highly used in neuroscience to discover biomarker candidates and also to study the differential expression of proteins at any given time in a proteome and they are then compared with the pattern of those from healthy ones.

Thus, to better understand the pathology based on secondary injury processes and plasticity, it is necessary to analyze entire spinal cord tissues in time, thus collecting tissues from the epicenter and both adjacent segments above (rostral) and below (caudal) the lesion firstly in acute, and afterwards in chronic SCI experimental models, expecting the release of different molecules. They will most likely reflect pathology *in situ*, at each specific segment, which may contribute to the final view of ascending or descending pathway disruption resulting in aggravation of clinical symptoms [41].

Nowadays, we can count on innovative proteomics technologies that can screen, identify image lipids and peptides in each spinal cord segment-derived conditioned medium (CM), or in the spinal cord tissue obtained *in vitro*, to better understand protein composition changes along the rostro-caudal axis after SCI with time in SCI.

Recently, application of shotgun proteomic analysis and label-free quantification to conditioned medium from the injured spinal cord (CM) identified chemokines (CXCL1; CXCL2; CXCL7, CCL2, CCL3, CCL22, CLCF1, and EMAP II) and neurotrophic factors (TGF, FGF-1, PDGF, and FGF1) in the lesion and rostral segments. These molecules are known to have immune-modulator and neurotrophic properties and ability to polarize macrophages/microglial cells into the M2 phenotype [10].

Chemokines are the most important molecules released immediately after SCI. Specific chemokines (CXCL1, CXCL2, CXCL3, CXCL5, CXCL7, CCL3, CCL20, and IL6) that are secreted by macrophages or epithelial cells after injury have the ability to attract neutrophils and lymphocytes, activate inflammation and stimulate extracellular matrix synthesis and tissue remodeling. Recent data showed that the cytokine profile changes in time between the segment above and below the lesion. This is in line with the hypothesis that immune cells that are attracted along the spinal cord upon injury insult are quite different between rostral (R1) and caudal (C1) segments in time. Recently, using proteomic analysis it has been documented that specific immune cells initially migrate toward R1 and then C1 segment [41]. In line with this,

IL6 and CCL20, which are known to attract T regulator lymphocytes through CCR6 binding, were expressed firstly in R1 at 3 days after SCI and secondly appeared in C1 at 7 days [40]. Furthermore, results from proteomic analysis were re-confirmed with cytokine/chemokine arrays and correlated with immunohistochemistry for neutrophils and Tregs. These experiments confirmed that neutrophils were abundantly detected in both R1 and C1 segments with a peak reached 3 days after SCI without any differences in terms of amount between each segment. However, their level decreased in time. In comparison, Tregs were present 3 days after SCI, in higher amounts in the rostral segment than in the caudal one. Their levels peak at 7 days for both segments and then decrease at 10 days [40]. These data are in line with the presence of CXCL1, CXCL3, CXCL5, CCL20, TIMP-1, and IL6 in R1 at 3 days, which are known to attract neutrophils and lymphocytes. In C1, a delay was observed in the recruitment of the Tregs, which were detected 7 days after SCI and correlated with the detection of CCL20 in C1 only at 7 days, whereas neutrophils and microglial cells were already present at 3 days [40]. Taken together, the results showed that C1 is clearly different from R1 in terms of cell types and molecular content in a time course manner, and is revealed to be a target segment for therapy.

The functionality of chemokine released from injured spinal cord tissue can be evaluated by chemotaxis assay, thus investigating the BV2 (microglial) cells activation, followed by Western blot, and M1/M2 polarization through CX3CR1 and CD206 expression.

In vitro chemotaxis assays confirmed that BV2 cells were highly responsive to the cytokine cocktail present in the CM from lesion and rostral sites, compared to CM from the caudal site after SCI. Interestingly, the BV2 migratory potency induced by CM derived from rostral and lesion segments was 37-fold higher compared to the ATP or LPS stimulations that increase their migration by close to 3-fold, due to the specific factors found in the complex CM [41, 42]. Furthermore, immunocytochemical studies prove that activated BV2 cells exposed to CM from the rostral segment overexpressed the CX3CR1 receptor, known to correspond with the M2 profile. This finding was strengthened by Western blot analysis and lack of labeling with C2KR, an M1 receptor [41]. These data together with *in vivo* CX3CR1 expression were in close coherence with published transcriptomic experiments showing that in the injured spinal cord, M2 gene expression is transiently expressed during 7 days after injury, while the M1 gene expression is maintained for up to 1 month [43].

Spatio-temporal proteomic analysis of spinal cord tissue between 3 and 10 days after injury provide clear evidence of regionalization between the rostral and caudal axes, with an expression of neurotrophic and immune modulatory factors in the rostral region, in contrast to inflammatory and apoptotic molecules in the caudal region.

Neutrophic factors were found at 3 and 7 days after injury and disappeared at 10 days. They were replaced by synaptogenesis factors reflecting the fact that a neurorepair process is taking place in the rostral segment after 10 days. In fact, more neurotrophic factors have been detected in the lesion and rostral parts, i.e., CTGF (connective tissue growth factor), NOV (Protein NOV homolog), PlGF (placenta growth factor), FGF-1 (fibroblast growth factor 1), BMP 2 or BMP3 (bone morphogenetic proteins (2 or 3), NGF, PGF, TGF beta (1–3) (transforming growth factor beta), periostin, GAP-43, neurotrimin, neurofascin, and hepatocyte growth factor-regulated tyrosine kinase substrate (HGS). In addition, molecules involved in neuronal development/differentiation/ neuronal migration, i.e., CRIP1 (cysteine-rich protein 1), DRP-5 (dihydropyrimidinase-related protein 5), Negr1 (neuronal growth regulator 1), NCAN (neurocan core protein), CD44, Wnt8, syndecan-4, nexin, and Bcl-2, were identified. Specific factors involved in immune cell chemotaxis or cellular adhesion, including complement factors (C1qb, C1qc, factor D, factor I, and CD59), tetraspanins (CD9 and CD82), and CD14 have also been characterized [40, 41].

In contrast, proteins produced in the caudal region were related to necrosis factors (BAX, BAD, Caspase 6, and neogenin), cytoskeleton proteins, synaptic vesicle exocytosis, chemoattractant factors, and neuronal postsynaptic density.

These data are in line with our previous *in vivo* results demonstrating that neurite outgrowth takes place from rostral to lesion but never in the opposite direction from caudal to the lesion. Furthermore, the presence of chemokines, lectins, and growth factors in the rostral but not in the caudal segment clearly document the immediate inflammatory response together with activity-dependent factors released by neurons and glia.

In order to investigate the neurotrophic role of CM derived from the injured tissue, studies testing neurite outgrowth in rat DRG explants have been undertaken. Data from these experiments confirmed that enhanced neurite sprouting of DRGs facilitated by CM from rostral and lesion segments were most likely mediated by the content of neurotrophic factors, i.e., FGF-1, NGF, PGF, BMP 2 or BMP3, GAP-43, neurotrimin, neurofascin, and other molecules involved in neuronal development/differentiation/migration. Although the principal role of NGF/TrkA pathways in sensory axon outgrowth has been widely demonstrated, other neurotrophic factors including the BMPs (members of the TGFβ superfamily) or GAP-43 have to be taken into account [41, 44].

In summary, it has been demonstrated that few days after SCI, a clear regionalization occurs between the rostral and caudal axes, with expression of neurotrophic and immunomodulatory factors in the rostral region, in contrast to inflammatory and apoptotic molecules in the caudal region. These data indicate the importance of stimulating neurite sprouting at segments below the lesion by inhibiting inflammation and turning polarization of M1 cells to the M2 state, which could have a clear impact on neurorepair. Therefore, these findings should be taken into account when planning new treatment strategies.

3. Neuroprotection in the CNS

Neuroprotection is defined as a curative strategy against harmful biochemical and molecular lesions that, if left untreated, lead to CNS damage [29]. The main purpose is to protect the damaged area by modifying the pathophysiological cascade with the limitation of harmful processes at secondary damage. In particular, the objective is to save those cell populations that are not directly affected by the injury, but due to secondary processes will underlay delayed apoptosis [45, 46]. In this regard, the primary goal is to suppress secondary inflammatory processes, edema and hemorrhage, and excitotoxicity that expand from the lesion center above and below the lesion site and acts destructively on healthy cells. Neuroprotection is among the specific therapies used in CNS injuries [47].

One of the important concepts that have recently resonated is the use of neuroprotective strategies that are applied to the spinal cord in conjunction with clinically proven operative methods of decompression and reconstruction of the spine. This clearly indicates that early intervention on traumatic spinal cord injuries can significantly affect the prognosis of the disease [3]. Therefore, great attention has been paid to studies that deal with the optimal timing of surgical procedures for acute spinal cord injury [48]. Previous data suggest that patients undergoing surgical decompression within 24 h after spinal cord injury have a significantly better recovery prognosis [29]. Currently, a number of innovative neuroprotective strategies for acute spinal cord injuries are being tested and evaluated in randomized controlled trials. Experimental studies on animal models showing promising results, such as ChABC, minocycline, riluzole, granulocyte colony stimulating factor (G-CSF), are now being tested in clinical studies [2, 49]. Hypothermia induced by intravascular cooling infusion administered epidural or subcutaneously has achieved success during acute SCI treatment.

3.1. Pharmacotherapy

Pharmacotherapy is one of the most widespread forms of treating secondary damage that use a wide variety of different types of molecules to target specific secondary processes. These are comprised of anti-inflammatory or neurostimulating compounds such as, minocycline, neurotrophic factors (BDNF, GDNF, NGF, and erythropoietin), and molecules that alleviate regenerating axons from the inhibitory effects of extracellular matrix molecules.

In particular, chondroitinase ABC eliminate CSPG with the major component NG2 which inhibits the regeneration of damaged axons [50]. Nogo-neutralizing antibodies or blockers of the post-receptors components RhoA, are used to improve long-distance axon regeneration and sprouting [25]. Previous studies have identified Rho pathway as important to control the neuronal response after CNS injury. Therefore, a drug called Cethrin® that blocks activation of Rho is actually in phase I/IIa of clinical trials [48]. The most encouraging findings were observed in patients with cervical SCI, whereas patients with injuries at thoracic level received only modest neurological recovery. Although the patient numbers were small in this trial, the results obtained indicate some evidence of efficacy to enhance functional recovery and warrant further clinical trials [51].

3.2. Molecular therapies: chondroitinase ABC, minocycline, tacrolimus, riluzole

Chondroitinase ABC is a bacterial enzyme that reduces the inhibitory effect of CSPGs at the site of injury. In order to increase CNS regeneration, only chondroitinase ABC purified from Proteus vulgaris [52] should be delivered. The mechanism of action lies in removing GAG chains from the nuclear protein and converting them to unsaturated disaccharides [34]. These stimulate the release of growth factors and proteins attached to GAGs of CSPGs, thereby enabling their diffusion and interaction with neural cell receptors. ChABC has been shown to promote neuroprotection and neuroregeneration [53]. Experimental administration of ChABC after cervical SCI positively affects the branching of damaged and intact descending pathways around which increased accumulation of CSPGs and then inhibition of axonal growth occurs. The neuroprotective effect of ChABC has been described also for the hemisection of the spinal cord [50, 54], transection of dorsal columns [55], and after compression injury of the thoracic spinal cord and the peripheral nerve [56] or in adult rats with visual deficits [57].ChABC administration is often combined with other therapeutic elements such as LiCl or Schwann cell transplantation [58] that can trigger regeneration. On the other hand, axonal plasticity supported by histological analyses did not correlate with motor function improvements of hind limbs. A similar conclusion was obtained by a group led by Cafferty [59]. There are several explanations for the negative correlation between the growths of axons without functional enhancements.

3.2.1. Orientation and quantity of functional synaptic connections

Functional recovery is dependent on correct orientation of axons and their functional links to the target structure. In some studies, linearly oriented as well as disordered nerve fibers that regrow through the lesion in different directions have been observed. Theoretically, they might increase the plasticity of tissues, because they cover a broader area. On the other hand, disorganized nerve fibers are often losing functional links with the target structure [60].

3.2.2. The time required for the maturation of functional linkages

Another possible negative factor that influenced clinical outcome may be the short-term survival of experimental animals required for functional contact formations. The intensive regeneration process in human patients progresses for months or years, and it is therefore necessary to prolong the length of survival in experimental animals from 3 to 6 months.

3.2.3. Method of ChABC administration

The important factors that affect the efficiency of ChABC therapy are: (i) method of local delivery, (ii) dose, (iii) timing of therapy, and (iv) efficacy of ChABC, since it is a bacterial enzyme which loses its activity *in vivo*. Therefore, to ensure its activity, repeated intrathecal delivery of ChABC or thermostable ChABC should be considered.

The undesirable effects of ChABC delivery have been observed only in rare cases. They are often related to the immune response against the enzyme or to neoepitopes (cleavage products) that this bacterial enzyme forms. Despite the rare negative effects, ChABC broadly reorganizes extracellular matrix, changes cell adhesion and tissue diffusion, and stimulates the functional recovery of damaged CNS [38].

In summary, the results confirmed that early reduction of NG2 allows extracellular matrix reorganization, creating a favorable environment for the initial neuroprotective processes to enable significant regrowth of injured axons in the epicenter of damage. Experimental studies also demonstrate that in order to achieve a better neurological outcome, ChABC needs to be combined with other therapeutic approaches. These may increase the plasticity of the injured tissue, create an environment for the axon outgrowth of fibers, and navigate these fibers to the right direction for the creation of fully functional synaptic connections.

Minocycline is a second-generation, semisynthetic tetracycline that has been commonly used in the treatment of acne vulgaris in children, because of its antibiotic properties against both gram-positive and gram-negative bacteria. However, it has been shown that minocycline can exert a variety of biological actions that are independent of their anti-microbial activity, including anti-inflammatory and anti-apoptotic activities, inhibition of proteolysis, angiogenesis, and tumor metastasis. Minocycline reveals high lipid solubility [61] and therefore easily crosses the blood–brain barrier [62]. This drug has been shown to be beneficial in various experimental animal models of CNS diseases. Primary mechanisms of action lie on the inhibition of microglia activation, which would justify its potential effectiveness in the treatment of neuroinflammatory and/or neurodegenerative disorders [63]. Different *in vitro* studies have described minocycline's ability to block LPS-stimulated inflammatory cytokine secretion and Toll-like-receptor (TLR)-2 surface expression in the BV-2 cell line and on primary microglia isolated from the brains of adult mice. Minocycline also attenuated the mRNA expression of inflammatory genes, including IL-6, IL-1β, major histocompatibility complex (MHC) II, and TLR-2. In experimental models of SCI, minocycline delivery significantly improved the function and strength of both hindlimbs, reduced the gross lesion size in the spinal cord, and enhanced axonal sparing. Minocycline-treated rats showed decreased release of cytochrome c from the mitochondria, resulting in markedly enhanced long-term hindlimb locomotion [64]. In traumatic SCI, results [65] showed that both short and long-term treatment with minocycline had a neuroprotective effect on the spinal cord segments located rostral to the injury epicenter. Minocycline has also been shown to improve functional recovery after SCI through the inhibition of pro-nerve growth factor production by microglia, thereby reducing oligodendrocyte death and apoptosis after traumatic SCI. It has been shown to inhibit the expression of p75 neurotrophin receptor and the activation of the Ras homolog gene family, member A (RhoA) after SCI [61]. Furthermore, previous study reported that minocycline might also exert a neuroprotective effect in SCI by inhibiting caspase expression and matrix metalloproteinases [65]. Metalloproteinases belong to a group of proteases that are responsible for the degradation and remodeling of the individual components of the intracellular matrix in normal tissue, and their activity is regulated by endogenous inhibitors. However, many pathological CNS conditions are characterized by increased metalloproteinase activity due to the reduced activity of their tissue inhibitors. The imbalance between intracellular matrix metalloproteinases and their inhibitors may lead to destructive proteolytic damage to the CNS tissue [45]. Minocycline has shown beneficial effects in many experimental studies [65] and was therefore also approved for phase I and II clinical trials in patients with completely injured spinal cord. The overall results confirmed the safety of the drug, but did not show improved motor outcomes in patients treated with minocycline compared to placebo. However, in a subset of patients with incomplete spinal cord injuries, patients experienced significant improvement [66]. Based on this promising outcome, a Phase III clinical trial was initiated in patients with acute spinal cord injury. This is currently ongoing and will be completed in 2018 [67].

Another interesting formulation is **FK506** (tacrolimus) isolated from the bacterium *Streptomyces tsukubaensis*, which presents a potent immunosuppressive drug. Primarily, it is used to reduce allograft rejection in organ transplantation, but also offers neuroprotective properties for central nervous system trauma. FK506 blocks the activation of calcineurin through the formation of complexes with immunophilins. However, it binds to a different immunophilin than cyclosporine A (CsA) [68]. FK506 has been found to increase nerve regeneration and functional re-innervation after peripheral nerve injury, as well as prevent axonal damage in toxic neuropathies [69]. Several studies document that FK506 delivery protects tissue from secondary injury and showed a beneficial effect during an acute SCI [70]. However, long-term administration of FK506 after experimental spinal cord injury in rats has shown to be not as effective [71]. FK506 was also used as a potent inhibitor of activated T-cells that infiltrates the injured spinal cord. Thus, it can modulate inflammation and ameliorate neuroprotection through its immunosuppressive action on immune cells [72]. Furthermore, the immunosuppressive action of FK506 was proven by the prevention of graft rejection following spinal cord ischemia and SCI [44].

Riluzole is commonly used in the treatment of amyotrophic lateral sclerosis (ALS) to protect against nerve cell degeneration. The possible mechanism of action of riluzole is blocking sodium channels as well as glutamate excitotoxicity. The deleterious effect of glutamate overproduction during CNS damage can be reduced by both reducing the synthesis and preventing its release into the synaptic cleft. In the case of riluzole, its mechanism of action is most likely thought to be the reduction of glutamate synthesis and thereby its release into the presynaptic region of the neuron. In a recent study, 155 patients were randomized to riluzole treatment (100 mg/day) or to placebo. The patients were monitored for 12–21 months [48]. Survival was significantly longer in the riluzole-treated group compared to placebo-treated patients. The median survival time was 17.7 months for riluzole compared to 14.9 months for placebo [4]. Additionally, there was a significant improvement in motor function in patients with cervical SCI receiving 50 mg riluzole twice a day for 14 days after injury, compared to the control group [73].

4. Regeneration

Regenerative medicine is a dynamically developing area of medicine whose mission is to restore damaged tissue. Although different tissues and organs have different recovery capabilities, there are diseases and CNS injuries that have limited regeneration and, unfortunately, they cannot be treated by conventional therapies. One of the innovative regenerative medicinal approaches is the use of stem cells and biomaterial-based treatments in order to replace damaged tissue or to supplement missing trophic factors in various CNS diseases [3].

The twenty-first century resonates with the rapid development of regenerative medicine, where methods of isolation and processing of stem cells and the use of highly compatible biodegradable materials and nanotechnologies directed to the treatment of SCI patients has been improved [74]. However, successful cell therapy is influenced by various factors such as: (i) selection and processing of stem cells (adult, induced pluripotent stem cells), (ii) delivery strategies (local, systemic), (iii) dosage (single, continuous), and (iv) appropriate timing of administration (acute, chronic phase of SCI). Selection of stem cells is important for their compatibility with host tissue. For this reason, in clinical studies, stem cells obtained from the tissues of the patient are preferred. Autologous stem cell transplantation obtained from the bone marrow and adipose tissue of a patient is used in the treatment of hematopoietic diseases, in the regeneration of bone tissue and cartilage, and possibly also in spinal trauma [74]. At present, an autologous transplantation of the so-called induced pluripotent stem cells (iPKB) derived from adult somatic cell patients has also been considered. By new procedures, we can reprogram a fully differentiated somatic cell (fibroblast) toward a cell with primitive pluripotent origin that is derived into the desired cell population [75]. In other cases, allogenic stem cells that meet the compatibility criteria (ABO, HLA) may still be used, but patients must still receive immunosuppressive therapy for a lifetime. In addition, stem cells are a major tool for gene therapy when they can produce some trophic factors and other molecules that are necessary for the regeneration of injured nerve tissue.

Among different **mono-therapies**, more **complex cellular therapy** has reached considerable attention due to targeting multiple aims, such as bridging the cavities or cysts, replacing dead cells, and creating a favorable environment allowing axonal regeneration [76].

4.1. Regenerative approaches toward biomaterials

SCI results in cysts or cavities at the site of the lesion, which gradually expand in the caudal direction. From this point of view, cell therapy alone for such a progressive pathological process as SCI is insufficient. Therefore, it is recommended to combine the administration of stem cells with biodegradable biomaterials that fill the cavities. The main objective is to optimize mechanical properties, cell adhesion, and biodegradability of synthetic or natural materials and develop new methods to deliver cells to the lesion site. One of the most important features for the successful integration of the implant into damaged tissue of the spinal cord is its optimal mechanical strength. If the biomaterial is too rigid, it can cause compression of regenerating axons and the formation of additional secondary cavities between the implant and surrounding spinal tissue. Therefore, it is preferable to use an injectable biomaterial that can properly adapt to the lesion [63, 77].The stem cells with which the implant should colonize also require the presence of growth factors that help them to survive in the unfavorable environment of the injured spinal cord. Chen and his scientific group compared the regenerative capabilities of several biodegradable multichannel biomaterials with different mechanical properties that were colonized by Schwann cells and implanted into the spinal cord after transection [63]. Compared to the poly-caprolactone fumarate material, which had significantly higher compression modulus values, biomaterials based on hydrogels showed significantly smaller cavities and promoted material vascularization and Schwann cell infiltration [63].

The biomaterial has to be biocompatible; this depends on the properties of the surface of the material and its interactions with cells or proteins [78]. However, we have to be aware of non-specific inflammatory responses of the recipient to the foreign biomaterial, and its extent determines the rate of implant biocompatibility. Interestingly, the acute response of the immune system that is mediated by macrophages or dendritic cells can be neuroprotective and can promote CNS regeneration. Modulation of the inflammatory response by the type of biomaterial surface can therefore be an auxiliary tool for repair mechanisms of the tissue. In principle, the physical properties of biomaterials should simulate the extracellular environment of the central nervous system and thereby ensure the diffusion of neurotrophic factors. Interactions between biomaterial surface and living tissue are usually mediated by a layer of proteins. Most biomaterials have an optimized surface with bioactive molecules or oligopeptide sequences [77]. This guarantees the adhesion of specific cells or their parts (e.g., axons).

Biodegradable materials are more desirable than non-degradable ones. Their degradation is most often mediated by hydrolysis and enzymatic cleavage. The rate of degradation can be controlled by various factors, such as molecular weight and polymer structure, crosslinking, and use of copolymers [79]. Of course, degradation products must not cause any immune response and the rate of breakdown of the material must be appropriate to the formation of new tissue. Biomaterials that are used to regenerate nerve tissue usually degrade for weeks or months, depending on the axonal and vascular material growth. Degradation can take place by gradual erosion of the surface of the material while maintaining the structural integrity of the material or by the gradual breakdown of the material structures. The first method is more advantageous because the collapse of the material may stop the regeneration process.

Alginate materials are natural and have a significant role because most of them are biodegradable. This group of natural materials also includes collagen, methylcellulose, or hyaluronic acid-based materials. The disadvantage is their natural variability and the risk of immunogenicity. The implantation of lyophilized alginate into the cavity of newborn or young rats stimulated the growth of non-myelinated and myelinated fibers in the hydrogel [80], as well as the formation of functional neuronal connections that have been demonstrated. In another study, the optimal combination of EGF and bFGF was chosen routinely in conventional 2D cultures in order to obtain the desired amount of proliferating cells. The goal was to create a strong but reversible binding of both factors to alginate-sulfate [81], allowing their prolonged and sustained local presentation to neural progenitors in cell culture. This develops an active biomaterial that eliminates the need for external continuous growth factor substitution during cell culture. However, it is crucial to determine the optimal concentration of growth factors that could mimic similar concentrations of bFGF/EGF commonly used in the 2D system culture (10–20 ng/ml for each factor/3 days). In this case, the equilibrium binding constant of the selected factors on alginate-sulfate plays an important role. The initial concentration of both bFGF and EGF factors (200 ng) was shown to be sufficient for their continuous release over 21-day incubation [82]. The concentration of growth factors released within the first week *in vitro* initiated cell proliferation and the formation of typical 3D neurospheres. Consequently, there was a decline in the growth factor concentrations; the cells migrated from the neurosphere and differentiated to neurons, astrocytes and oligodendrocytes. These results confirmed that the 3D alginate biomaterial, which gradually released growth factors, creates optimal conditions for long-term survival and differentiation of neural progenitors *in vitro* [82].

The developed 3D biomaterial was implanted locally into SCI rats. The results confirmed that the optimal bioavailability of growth factors (EGF and bFGF) from the implant stimulated neuroregenerative processes. Enhanced sparing of spinal cord tissue and increased number of surviving neurons (ChAT-cholinacetyltransferase-positive neurons), corticospinal fibers (BDA-labeled), and blood vessels at the site of injury [83] occurred. Inflammatory processes were partially suppressed, but not astrogliosis. These partial results indicate the possible use of active alginate biomaterials enriched with bioactive molecules in the treatment of CNS trauma [83].

Although the biomaterials themselves can affect nerve tissue regeneration by creating a space for cell growth through the lesion, it is increasingly clear that combined therapy has a synergistic effect and leads to better results. Therefore, biomaterials are most often combined with different types of cells or enzymes digesting proteoglycans in glial scars, as known for chondroitinase ABC. The most commonly used cells are MSC, Schwann cells, and neural stem cells that can express Noggin, promoting neurogenesis and suppressing gliogenesis [84]. Biomaterials can also serve to release the biologically active substance, which can then create a gradient that promotes cell growth into the implant. Biologically active agents may be growth factors (EGF, FGF), cytokines, neurotrophins (NT3, NGF, BDNF, and GDNF), neurotransmitters, and anti-axon growth inhibitory antibodies [85].

In conclusion, it is necessary to combine these strategies to further enhance the final effect.

Acknowledgements

Supported by APVV 15-0613, ERANET- AxonRepair, INSERM U1003, VEGA 2/0125/15, SK-FR-2015-0018/ Stefanik, EU SF ITMS 26240220008.

Author details

Dasa Cizkova[1,2,3]*, Adriana-Natalia Murgoci[1,2,3], Lenka Kresakova[1], Katarina Vdoviakova[1], Milan Cizek[1], Tomas Smolek[3], Veronika Cubinkova[3], Jusal Quanico[2], Isabelle Fournier[2] and Michel Salzet[2]

*Address all correspondence to: cizkova.dasa@gmail.com

1 University of Veterinary Medicine and Pharmacy in Kosice, Slovakia

2 Laboratoire Protéomique, Réponse Inflammatoire et Spectrométrie de Masse (PRISM), Université Lille 1, Lille, France

3 Institute of Neuroimmunology, Slovak Academy of Sciences, Bratislava, Slovakia

References

[1] Munce SE, Straus SE, Fehlings MG, Voth J, Nugaeva N, Jang E, Webster F, Jaglal SB. Impact of psychological characteristics in self-management in individuals with traumatic spinal cord injury. Spinal Cord. 2015;**54**(1):29-33

[2] Nagoshi N, Fehlings MG. Investigational drugs for the treatment of spinal cord injury: Review of preclinical studies and evaluation of clinical trials from Phase I to II. Expert Opinion on Investigational Drugs. 2015a;**24**(5):645-658

[3] Siddiqui AM, Khazaei M, Fehlings MG. Translating mechanisms of neuroprotection, regeneration, and repair to treatment of spinal cord injury. Progress in Brain Research. 2015; **218**:15-54

[4] Nagoshi N, Nakashima H, Fehlings MG. Riluzole as a neuroprotective drug for spinal cord injury: From bench to bedside. Molecules. 2015b;**20**(5):7775-7789

[5] Donnelly DJ, Popovich PG. Inflammation and its role in neuroprotection, axonal regeneration and functional recovery after spinal cord injury. Experimental Neurology. 2008; **209**(2):378-388

[6] Schwab ME. Repairing the injured spinal cord. Science. 2002;**295**(5557):1029-1031

[7] Ransohoff RM, Liu L, Cardona AE. Chemokines and chemokine receptors: Multipurpose players in neuroinflammation. International Review of Neurobiology. 2007;**82**: 187-204

[8] Kreutzberg GW. Microglia: A sensor for pathological events in the CNS. Trends in Neurosciences. 1996;**19**(8):312-318

[9] Aguzzi A, Barres BA, Bennett ML. Microglia: Scapegoat, saboteur, or something else? Science. 2013;**339**(6116):156-161

[10] Fitch MT, Silver J. CNS injury, glial scars, and inflammation: Inhibitory extracellular matrices and regeneration failure. Experimental Neurology. 2008;**209**(2):294-301

[11] Aloisi F. Immune function of microglia. GLIA. 2001;**36**(2):165-179

[12] Means ED, Anderson DK. Neuronophagia by leukocytes in experimental spinal cord injury. Journal of Neuropathology and Experimental Neurology. 1983;**42**(6):707-719

[13] Tonai T, Shiba K, Taketani Y, Ohmoto Y, Murata K, Muraguchi M, Ohsaki H, Takeda E, Nishisho T. A neutrophil elastase inhibitor (ONO-5046) reduces neurologic damage after spinal cord injury in rats. Journal of Neurochemistry. 2001;**78**(5):1064-1072

[14] Taoka Y, Okajima K, Uchiba M, Murakami K, Kushimoto S, Johno M, Naruo M, Okabe H, Takatsuki K. Role of neutrophils in spinal cord injury in the rat. Neuroscience. 1997;**79**(4):1177-1182

[15] McDonald PP, Bald A, Cassatella MA. Activation of the NF-kappaB pathway by inflammatory stimuli in human neutrophils. Blood. 1997;**89**(9):3421-3433

[16] McDonald PP, Cassatella MA. Activation of transcription factor NF-kappa B by phagocytic stimuli in human neutrophils. FEBS Letters. 1997;**412**(3):583-586

[17] Cassatella MA. The production of cytokines by polymorphonuclear neutrophils. Immunology Today. 1995;**16**(1):21-26

[18] Sica A, Schioppa T, Mantovani A, Allavena P. Tumour-associated macrophages are a distinct M2 polarised population promoting tumour progression: Potential targets of anti-cancer therapy. European Journal of Cancer. 2006;**42**(6):717-727

[19] De Wit J, De Winter F, Klooster J, Verhaagen J. Semaphorin 3A displays a punctate distribution on the surface of neuronal cells and interacts with proteoglycans in the extracellular matrix. Molecular and Cellular Neurosciences. 2005;**29**(1):40-55

[20] Biber K, Boddeke E, Neuronal CC. Chemokines: The distinct roles of CCL21 and CCL2 in neuropathic pain. Frontiers in Cellular Neuroscience. 2014;**8**:210

[21] Chavarria A, Cardenas G. Neuronal influence behind the central nervous system regulation of the immune cells. Frontiers in Integrative Neuroscience. 2013;**7**:64

[22] Liu WL, Lee YH, Tsai SY, Hsu CY, Sun YY, Yang LY, Tsai SH, Yang WC. Methylprednisolone inhibits the expression of glial fibrillary acidic protein and chondroitin sulfate proteoglycans in reactivated astrocytes. GLIA. 2008;**56**(13):1390-1400

[23] Eddleston M, Mucke L. Molecular profile of reactive astrocytes—Implications for their role in neurologic disease. Neuroscience. 1993;**54**(1):15-36

[24] Fawcett JW, Asher RA. The glial scar and central nervous system repair. Brain Research Bulletin. 1999;**49**(6):377-391

[25] Schwab ME. Nogo and axon regeneration. Current Opinion in Neurobiology. 2004;**14**(1): 118-124

[26] Schwab ME. Myelin-associated inhibitors of neurite growth and regeneration in the CNS. Trends in Neurosciences. 1990;**13**(11):452-456

[27] Wang KC, Koprivica V, Kim JA, Sivasankaran R, Guo Y, Neve RL, He Z. Oligodendrocyte-myelin glycoprotein is a Nogo receptor ligand that inhibits neurite outgrowth. Nature. 2002;**417**(6892):941-944

[28] Cai D, Shen Y, De Bellard M, Tang S, Filbin MT. Prior exposure to neurotrophins blocks inhibition of axonal regeneration by MAG and myelin via a cAMP-dependent mechanism. Neuron. 1999;**22**(1):89-101

[29] Fawcett JW, Curt A, Steeves JD, Coleman WP, Tuszynski MH, Lammertse D, Bartlett PF, Blight AR, Dietz V, Ditunno J, Dobkin BH, Havton LA, Ellaway PH, Fehlings MG, Privat A, Grossman R, Guest JD, Kleitman N, Nakamura M, Gaviria M, Short D. Guidelines for the conduct of clinical trials for spinal cord injury as developed by the ICCP panel: Spontaneous recovery after spinal cord injury and statistical power needed for thera-peutic clinical trials. Spinal Cord. 2007;**45**(3):190-205

[30] Bradbury EJ, McMahon SB. Spinal cord repair strategies: Why do they work? Nature Reviews. Neuroscience. 2006;**7**(8):644-653

[31] Tang X, Davies JE, Davies SJ. Changes in distribution, cell associations, and protein expression levels of NG2, neurocan, phosphacan, brevican, versican V2, and tenascin-C during acute to chronic maturation of spinal cord scar tissue. Journal of Neuroscience Research. 2003;**71**(3):427-444

[32] Bandtlow CE, Zimmermann DR. Proteoglycans in the developing brain: New concep-tual insights for old proteins. Physiological Reviews. 2000;**80**(4):1267-1290

[33] Grumet M, Milev P, Sakurai T, Karthikeyan L, Bourdon M, Margolis RK, Margolis RU. Interactions with tenascin and differential effects on cell adhesion of neurocan and phos-phacan, two major chondroitin sulfate proteoglycans of nervous tissue. The Journal of Biological Chemistry. 1994;**269**(16):12142-12146

[34] Deepa SS, Yamada S, Zako M, Goldberger O, Sugahara K. Chondroitin sulfate chains on syndecan-1 and syndecan-4 from normal murine mammary gland epithelial cells are structurally and functionally distinct and cooperate with heparan sulfate chains to bind growth factors. A novel function to control binding of midkine, pleiotrophin, and basic fibroblast growth factor. The Journal of Biological Chemistry. 2004;**279**(36):37368-37376

[35] Dawson MR, Levine JM, Reynolds R. NG2-expressing cells in the central nervous sys-tem: Are they oligodendroglial progenitors? Journal of Neuroscience Research. 2000; **61**(5):471-479

[36] Bu J, Akhtar N, Nishiyama A. Transient expression of the NG2 proteoglycan by a sub-population of activated macrophages in an excitotoxic hippocampal lesion. GLIA. 2001; **34**(4):296-310

[37] Hall A, Giese NA, Richardson WD. Spinal cord oligodendrocytes develop from ventrally derived progenitor cells that express PDGF alpha-receptors. Development. 1996; **122**(12):4085-4094

[38] Novotna I, Slovinska L, Vanicky I, Cizek M, Radonak J, Cizkova D. IT delivery of ChABC modulates NG2 and promotes GAP-43 axonal regrowth after spinal cord injury. Cellular and Molecular Neurobiology. 2011;**31**(8):1129-1139

[39] Jones LL, Yamaguchi Y, Stallcup WB, Tuszynski MH. NG2 is a major chondroitin sulfate proteoglycan produced after spinal cord injury and is expressed by macrophages and oligodendrocyte progenitors. The Journal of Neuroscience. 2002;**22**(7):2792-2803

[40] Devaux S, Cizkova D, Quanico J, Franck J, Nataf S, Pays L, Hauberg-Lotte L, Maass P, Kobarg JH, Kobeissy F, Meriaux C, Wisztorski M, Slovinska L, Blasko J, Cigankova V, Fournier I, Salzet M. Proteomic analysis of the spatio-temporal based molecular kinetics of acute spinal cord injury identifies a time- and segment-specific window for effective tissue repair. Molecular & Cellular Proteomics. 2016;**15**(8):2641-2670

[41] Cizkova D, Le Marrec-Croq F, Franck J, Slovinska L, Grulova I, Devaux S, Lefebvre C, Fournier I, Salzet M. Alterations of protein composition along the rostro-caudal axis after spinal cord injury: Proteomic, *in vitro* and *in vivo* analyses. Frontiers in Cellular Neuroscience. 2014;**8**:105

[42] Rahmat Z, Jose S, Ramasamy R, Vidyadaran S. Reciprocal interactions of mouse bone marrow-derived mesenchymal stem cells and BV2 microglia following lipopolysaccharide stimulation. Stem Cell Research & Therapy. 2013;**4**(1):12

[43] Kigerl KA, Gensel JC, Ankeny DP, Alexander JK, Donnelly DJ, Popovich PG. Identification of two distinct macrophage subsets with divergent effects causing either neurotoxicity or regeneration in the injured mouse spinal cord. The Journal of Neuroscience. 2009; **29**(43):13435-13444

[44] Cizkova D, Kakinohana O, Kucharova K, Marsala S, Johe K, Hazel T, Hefferan MP, Marsala M. Functional recovery in rats with ischemic paraplegia after spinal grafting of human spinal stem cells. Neuroscience. 2007;**147**(2):546-560

[45] Fleming JC, Norenberg MD, Ramsay DA, Dekaban GA, Marcillo AE, Saenz AD, Pasquale-Styles M, Dietrich WD, Weaver LC. The cellular inflammatory response in human spinal cords after injury. Brain. 2006;**129**(Pt 12):3249-3269

[46] Norenberg MD, Smith J, Marcillo A. The pathology of human spinal cord injury: Defining the problems. Journal of Neurotrauma. 2004;**21**(4):429-440

[47] Ahn H, Bailey CS, Rivers CS, Noonan VK, Tsai EC, Fourney DR, Attabib N, Kwon BK, Christie SD, Fehlings MG, Finkelstein J, Hurlbert RJ, Townson A, Parent S, Drew B, Chen J, Dvorak MF. Effect of older age on treatment decisions and outcomes among patients with traumatic spinal cord injury. CMAJ. 2015;**187**(12):873-880

[48] Fehlings MG, Nakashima H, Nagoshi N, Chow DS, Grossman RG, Kopjar B. Rationale, design and critical end points for the riluzole in acute spinal cord injury study (RISCIS):

A randomized, double-blinded, placebo-controlled parallel multi-center trial. Spinal Cord. 2015;**54**(1):8-15

[49] Fawcett JW. Overcoming inhibition in the damaged spinal cord. Journal of Neurotrauma. 2006;**23**(3-4):371-383

[50] Bradbury EJ, Moon LD, Popat RJ, King VR, Bennett GS, Patel PN, Fawcett JW, McMahon SB. Chondroitinase ABC promotes functional recovery after spinal cord injury. Nature. 2002;**416**(6881):636-640

[51] Fehlings MG, Theodore N, Harrop J, Maurais G, Kuntz C, Shaffrey CI, Kwon BK, Chapman J, Yee A, Tighe A, McKerracher L. A phase I/IIa clinical trial of a recombinant Rho protein antagonist in acute spinal cord injury. Journal of Neurotrauma. 2011;**28**(5):787-796

[52] Yamagata T, Saito H, Habuchi O, Suzuki S. Purification and properties of bacterial chondroitinases and chondrosulfatases. The Journal of Biological Chemistry. 1968;**243**(7): 1523-1535

[53] Rolls A, Avidan H, Cahalon L, Schori H, Bakalash S, Litvak V, Lev S, Lider O, Schwartz M. A disaccharide derived from chondroitin sulphate proteoglycan promotes central nervous system repair in rats and mice. The European Journal of Neuroscience. 2004;**20**(8): 1973-1983

[54] Caggiano AO, Zimber MP, Ganguly A, Blight AR, Gruskin EA. Chondroitinase ABCI improves locomotion and bladder function following contusion injury of the rat spinal cord. Journal of Neurotrauma. 2005;**22**(2):226-239

[55] Massey JM, Hubscher CH, Wagoner MR, Decker JA, Amps J, Silver J, Onifer SM. Chondroitinase ABC digestion of the perineuronal net promotes functional collateral sprouting in the cuneate nucleus after cervical spinal cord injury. The Journal of Neuroscience. 2006;**26**(16):4406-4414

[56] Galtrey CM, Asher RA, Nothias F, Fawcett JW. Promoting plasticity in the spinal cord with chondroitinase improves functional recovery after peripheral nerve repair. Brain. 2007;**130**(Pt 4):926-939

[57] Pizzorusso T, Medini P, Landi S, Baldini S, Berardi N, Maffei L. Structural and functional recovery from early monocular deprivation in adult rats. Proceedings of the National Academy of Sciences of the United States of America. 2006;**103**(22):8517-8522

[58] Chau CH, Shum DK, Li H, Pei J, Lui YY, Wirthlin L, Chan YS, Xu XM. Chondroitinase ABC enhances axonal regrowth through Schwann cell-seeded guidance channels after spinal cord injury. The FASEB Journal. 2004;**18**(1):194-196

[59] Cafferty WB, Bradbury EJ, Lidierth M, Jones M, Duffy PJ, Pezet S, McMahon SB. Chondroitinase ABC-mediated plasticity of spinal sensory function. The Journal of Neuroscience. 2008;**28**(46):11998-12009

[60] Bradbury EJ, Carter LM. Manipulating the glial scar: Chondroitinase ABC as a therapy for spinal cord injury. Brain Research Bulletin. 2011;**84**(4-5):306-316

[61] Yune TY, Lee JY, Jung GY, Kim SJ, Jiang MH, Kim YC, Oh YJ, Markelonis GJ, Oh TH. Minocycline alleviates death of oligodendrocytes by inhibiting pro-nerve growth factor production in microglia after spinal cord injury. The Journal of Neuroscience. 2007; **27**(29):7751-7761

[62] Kwon BK, Fisher CG, Dvorak MF, Tetzlaff W. Strategies to promote neural repair and regeneration after spinal cord injury. Spine (Phila Pa 1976). 2005;**30**(17 Suppl):S3-13

[63] Chen BK, Knight AM, de Ruiter GC, Spinner RJ, Yaszemski MJ, Currier BL, Windebank AJ. Axon regeneration through scaffold into distal spinal cord after transection. Journal of Neurotrauma. 2009;**26**(10):1759-1771

[64] Teng YD, Choi H, Onario RC, Zhu S, Desilets FC, Lan S, Woodard EJ, Snyder EY, Eichler ME, Friedlander RM. Minocycline inhibits contusion-triggered mitochondrial cytochrome c release and mitigates functional deficits after spinal cord injury. Proceedings of the National Academy of Sciences of the United States of America. 2004;**101**(9):3071-3076

[65] Saganova K, Orendacova J, Cizkova D, Vanicky I. Limited minocycline neuroprotection after balloon-compression spinal cord injury in the rat. Neuroscience Letters. 2008; **433**(3):246-249

[66] Monaco EA 3rd, Weiner GM, Friedlander RM. Randomized-controlled trial of minocycline for spinal cord injury shows promise. Neurosurgery. 2013;**72**(2):N17-N19

[67] Ahuja CS, Fehlings M. Concise review: Bridging the gap: Novel neuroregenerative and neuroprotective strategies in spinal cord injury. Stem Cells Translational Medicine. 2016; **5**(7):914-924

[68] Powell JD, Zheng Y. Dissecting the mechanism of T-cell anergy with immunophilin ligands. Current Opinion in Investigational Drugs. 2006;**7**(11):1002-1007

[69] Udina E, Ceballos D, Verdu E, Gold BG, Navarro X. Bimodal dose-dependence of FK506 on the rate of axonal regeneration in mouse peripheral nerve. Muscle & Nerve. 2002; **26**(3):348-355

[70] Madsen JR, MacDonald P, Irwin N, Goldberg DE, Yao GL, Meiri KF, Rimm IJ, Stieg PE, Benowitz LI. Tacrolimus (FK506) increases neuronal expression of GAP-43 and improves functional recovery after spinal cord injury in rats. Experimental Neurology. 1998; **154**(2):673-683

[71] Saganova K, Orendacova J, Sulla I Jr, Filipcik P, Cizkova D, Vanicky I. Effects of long-term FK506 administration on functional and histopathological outcome after spinal cord injury in adult rat. Cellular and Molecular Neurobiology. 2009;**29**(6-7):1045-1051

[72] Ankeny DP, Popovich PG. Mechanisms and implications of adaptive immune responses after traumatic spinal cord injury. Neuroscience. 2009;**158**(3):1112-1121

[73] Karadimas SK, Laliberte AM, Tetreault L, Chung YS, Arnold P, Foltz WD, Fehlings MG. Riluzole blocks perioperative ischemia-reperfusion injury and enhances postdecompression outcomes in cervical spondylotic myelopathy. Science Translational Medicine. 2015;**7**(316):316ra194

[74] Sykova E, Jendelova P, Urdzikova L, Lesny P, Hejcl A. Bone marrow stem cells and polymer hydrogels—Two strategies for spinal cord injury repair. Cellular and Molecular Neurobiology. 2006;**26**(7-8):1113-1129

[75] Takahashi K, Yamanaka S. Induction of pluripotent stem cells from mouse embryonic and adult fibroblast cultures by defined factors. Cell. 2006;**126**(4):663-676

[76] Rowland JW, Hawryluk GW, Kwon B, Fehlings MG. Current status of acute spinal cord injury pathophysiology and emerging therapies: Promise on the horizon. Neurosurgical Focus. 2008;**25**(5):E2

[77] Kubinova S, Horak D, Hejcl A, Plichta Z, Kotek J, Proks V, Forostyak S, Sykova E. SIKVAV-modified highly superporous PHEMA scaffolds with oriented pores for spinal cord injury repair. Journal of Tissue Engineering and Regenerative Medicine. 2015; **9**(11):1298-1309

[78] Fournier E, Passirani C, Montero-Menei CN, Benoit JP. Biocompatibility of implantable synthetic polymeric drug carriers: Focus on brain biocompatibility. Biomaterials. 2003; **24**(19):3311-3331

[79] Hu J, Kai D, Ye H, Tian L, Ding X, Ramakrishna S, Loh XJ. Electrospinning of poly(glycerol sebacate)-based nanofibers for nerve tissue engineering. Materials Science & Engineering. C, Materials for Biological Applications. 2017;**70**(Pt 2):1089-1094

[80] Kataoka K, Suzuki Y, Kitada M, Ohnishi K, Suzuki K, Tanihara M, Ide C, Endo K, Nishimura Y. Alginate, a bioresorbable material derived from brown seaweed, enhances elongation of amputated axons of spinal cord in infant rats. Journal of Biomedical Materials Research. 2001;**54**(3):373-384

[81] Freeman I, Kedem A, Cohen S. The effect of sulfation of alginate hydrogels on the specific binding and controlled release of heparin-binding proteins. Biomaterials. 2008; **29**(22):3260-3268

[82] Cizkova D, Slovinska L, Grulova I, Salzet M, Cikos S, Kryukov O, Cohen S. The influence of sustained dual-factor presentation on the expansion and differentiation of neural progenitors in affinity-binding alginate scaffolds. Journal of Tissue Engineering and Regenerative Medicine. 2013

[83] Grulova I, Slovinska L, Blasko J, Devaux S, Wisztorski M, Salzet M, Fournier I, Kryukov O, Cohen S, Cizkova D. Delivery of alginate scaffold releasing two trophic factors for spinal cord injury repair. Scientific Reports. 2015;**5**:13702

[84] Enzmann GU, Benton RL, Woock JP, Howard RM, Tsoulfas P, Whittemore SR. Consequences of noggin expression by neural stem, glial, and neuronal precursor cells engrafted into the injured spinal cord. Experimental Neurology. 2005;**195**(2):293-304

[85] Dodla MC, Bellamkonda RV. Differences between the effect of anisotropic and isotropic laminin and nerve growth factor presenting scaffolds on nerve regeneration across long peripheral nerve gaps. Biomaterials. 2008;**29**(1):33-46

6

In Vitro Models of Spinal Cord Injury

Lucia Slovinska, Juraj Blasko, Miriam Nagyova,
Eva Szekiova and Dasa Cizkova

Abstract

Living organisms are extremely complex functional systems. At present, there are many *in vivo* models of spinal cord injury (SCI) that allow the modeling of any type of central nervous system (CNS) injury, however, with some disadvantages. The production of injury models can be a highly invasive and time-consuming process and requires high technical requirements, and costly financial issues should also be taken into account. Of course, a large number of animals have been used to obtain the relevant data of statistical significance. All of these aspects can be reduced by carrying out experiments in *in vitro* conditions. The primary advantage of *in vitro* method is that it simplifies the system under study. There are two major groups of *in vitro* model in use: cell culture and organotypic slice (OTS) culture. OTS is an intermediate system of the screening of *in vitro* cell culture and animal models and represents the *in vitro* system preserving the basic tissue architecture that able to closely mimic the cellular and physiological characteristics *in vivo*. *In vitro* models are the preferred methods for the study of acute or subacute pathophysiology after a trauma stimulus, enabling precise control on the extracellular environment, easy and repeatable access to the cells.

Keywords: *in vitro* model, spinal cord injury (SCI), cell culture, co-culture, organotypic slice (OTS) culture

1. Introduction

Spinal cord injury (SCI) is a critical incurable difficulty affecting the quality of life of patients and society equally. The spinal cord injury interferes predominantly with motor function defects, which substantially restrict normal daily activities, thus leading to serious psychological trauma. Today, the majority of patients are left paralyzed with unsuccessful treat-ment currently available. Many strategies, including surgical, transplantations, pharmacological, neurophysiological, and others approaches, have been used and examined in attempts to develop new and successful therapies that will allow patients to get the valuable life they lived before the injury [1].

First, before devising a new treatment for spinal cord injury, it is also important to know the processes of nerve tissue regeneration, neurogenesis, and gliogenesis, which can be influenced in many ways. The answer to these needs, a growing number of animal models have been introduced and utilized. The creation of *in vivo* injury models requires many invasive inter-ventions and is time consuming. The financial costs of such models as well as technical equipment are often high. However, the biggest problem of the *in vivo* models is the utilization of large amounts of experimental animals. All of these facts can be reduced by carrying out experiments in *in vitro* conditions. *In vitro* experimental models are needed to understand the cellular mechanisms and pathophysiology of the injured spinal cord (SC) and to provide evidence for further treatment. This is also the right place to mention the principles of the 3Rs (Replacement, Reduction, and Refinement). The principles of the 3Rs were developed as a framework for humane animal research and became embedded in national and international legislation regulating the use of animals in scientific procedures in most world countries. There are two major groups of *in vitro* model in use: cell culture and organotypic slice (OTS) culture.

2. Cell cultures

After central nervous system (CNS) injury, the acute primary and the chronic secondary damage takes place. After initial mechanical insult, a rapid deformation of CNS tissue happens, causing an immediate cell death in the epicenter of injury site followed by a cascade of processes leading to the secondary damage. Traumatic injury disrupts spinal white matter tracts resulting in the loss of sensory and motor function. This loss of function is generally permanent due to the limited regenerative capacity of the CNS [2]. Cells used for *in vitro* modeling should have morphological, functional qualities, and relevant requirements depending on disease, injury, and ultimate goal of the proposed experiments. The commonly used *in vitro* cell culture models of SCI include:

i.   Primary isolated cells, neurons, oligodendrocytes, astrocytes, or microglia cells [3, 4]. Primary cells are obtained from the dissociated neural tissues, spinal cord, or brain and are usually cultivated immediately after the isolation as "primo-cultures." The origin of these cells could be embryonal, fetal, neonatal, or adult [5, 6]. It is well known that younger cells are more potent according to their strong proliferative activity, in contrary to terminally differentiated poor proliferating capacity owning adult cells [6]. By using the primary cultures, we can investigate the behavior and intercommu-nication of the individual or mixed cell populations. These populations preserve the main characteristics similar to the *in vivo* examined types of cells [7]. Very often used are also the immortalized cell lines, which are in fact the primary cells with genetical modification.

ii.   Co-culture of neuronal cells with different cell types, which are present in the glial
             scar [8, 9]. *In vitro* cultures offer simplified, high throughput systems to study disease,
             drug toxicity, and biological processes by controlling environmental factors and
             directly measuring cell responses [10].

2.1. *In vitro* model of glial scar

The characteristic manifestation of the secondary reactive phase is scar formation at the initial
impact site, which represents the major obstruction to CNS regeneration. The glial scar is rich
in different cells (microglia and reactive astrocytes), myelin-associated inhibitors, and it
physically surrounds the damaged tissue. To study the components of the glial scar, many
models of co-cultivation of neurons with others glial scar situated cells have been developed
[8, 9, 11]. By combining two pivotal aspects of CNS damage, mechanical injury and co-
cultivation with meningeal cells in *in vitro* scar formation model, it has been shown that
astrocytes increase the expression of GFAP (glial fibrillary acidic protein), as well as the scar-
associated markers, e.g., phosphacan, neurocan, and tenascin. Subsequent short-time co-
cultivation with different developmental neuronal populations led to significantly reduced
neurite growth in this scar-like model [9]. After spinal cord injury, demyelination of spared
white matter significantly hinders spontaneous function recovery [12]. To understand the
processes related to this phenomenon, a wide range of developed cultures in which the many
stages of myelination can be followed over time are used [13–15]. These myelinating cultures
involve plating dissociated rat spinal cord cells onto a confluent monolayer of neurosphere-
derived astrocytes. Sorensen et al. [16] compared the different types of cells in the process of
myelination promotion of CNS axons. The mixed cell population of dissociated embryonal
spinal cord was cultivated on olfactory ensheathing cells (OECs), Schwann cells (SchCs), or
neurosphere-derived astrocytes to study the mutual interactions in context to affect the
myelination. Myelin internodes and nodes of Ranvier were often found only in the cells
cultivated onto neurosphere-derived astrocytes. This model is very useful to investigate the
CNS axonal myelination because it recapitulates the processes occurring in CNS *in vivo*. On
the basis of these cultures, it has been shown that astrocytes have a direct role in promoting
myelination either by releasing a soluble factor or by cell–cell contact [16]. Also, the phenotype
of astrocytes has a crucial role in determining their effects on myelination. Myelination is poor
when the myelinating cultures are plated on quiescent astrocytes but enhanced when they are
plated on a more reactive/activated phenotype. Interestingly, quiescent astrocytes secreted
CXCL10, which did not appear to directly affect the purified oligodendrocyte progenitor cell
differentiation but had the effect on the ability of oligodendrocytes to ensheath axons [13].
Astrocytes exhibit dynamic cell process movement and changes in their membrane topogra-
phy as they interact with axons and oligodendrocytes during the process of myelination [15].
These observations may have important implications with respect to the development of
therapeutic strategies to promote CNS remyelination in demyelinating diseases. Also other
models have been developed to investigate and to understand the molecular mechanisms of
CNS axon regeneration. The process of axon regeneration can be monitored by neurite
outgrowth assays, which often represent the phenotypic expression of regeneration progress.
In neurite outgrowth assays, the neurons are cultivated on an adherent substrate, and the

neurite growth is evaluated in specific medium conditions for extended periods of time, and then the overall length of the radial outgrowth is measured. Primary neurons (neurons derived from dorsal roots ganglion, cerebellum, cortex, or hippocampus) are considered more biologically relevant to neurons *in vivo* instead of induced pluripotent stem cells or any special cell lines [17].

2.2 *In vitro*

The majority of SCI occurring in human is due to the compression of spinal cord; therefore most *in vitro* models have been designed to mimic this type of injury. To simulate the spinal cord injury *in vitro*, the confluent layer of astrocytes and dissociated embryonic spinal cord cells plated onto them are cut with scalpel blade, the so-called scratch model. Such treatment creates an empty area without any cells—lesion. With an increasing time of cultivation, the situation around the injury becomes comparable to the SCI *in vivo*. The microglial cells and astrocytes start to migrate to the injury site. Conversely, the decrease in neurite density and the process of demyelination start as the consequences of disrupting confluent cell layer. The main purpose of this model is to find out, to recognize any factors, molecules, biomaterials, even cells that can contribute, may be, to accelerate the potential regeneration of remaining cells destroyed by injury. The closure of this lesion could be modified using different Rho/ ROCK inhibitors [11] or by cAMP modulators, which promote neurite outgrowth and myelination [5]. *In vitro* models are the preferred methods for the study of acute or sub-acute pathophysiology after a trauma stimulus enabling the precise control of the extracellular environment, easy and repeatable access to the cells.

To imitate the SCI in our experimental model, the P1 rat spinal cord cells were mechanically scratched across the cell monolayer with a pipette tip. The result of this handling was the linear cell-free area/lesion which varied between 400 - 600 μm in width. After washing out the scraped cells with PBS (phosphate-buffered saline), cells were maintained for up to 10 days in culture. During the cultivation time, the cultures remained viable. Cell migration or wound closure of the scratched surface was observed and photographed at daily intervals. To investigate the potential stimulative effect of mesenchymal stem cells (MSCs) on the neural cells, we treated such injured cultures with conditioned medium obtained from rat bone marrow MSCs. In fact, MSCs cannot differentiate into fully functional neurons, or into others neural cells; the supporting effect of neuroregeneration and neuroprotection is mediated by specific neurotro-phic factors and cytokines produced by MSCs [18]. All experiments conformed to the Slovak Law for Animal Protection No. 377/2012 and 436/2012 transposed from the European Com-munities Council Directive (2010/63/EU) and were approved by the Institutional Ethical Committee for animal research. Our preliminary data showed that the cell-free area in injured group treated with MSC conditioned medium became filled with reactive astrocytes, microglia cells, and oligodendrocyte in a shorter time when compared to untreated controls (**Figure 1**).

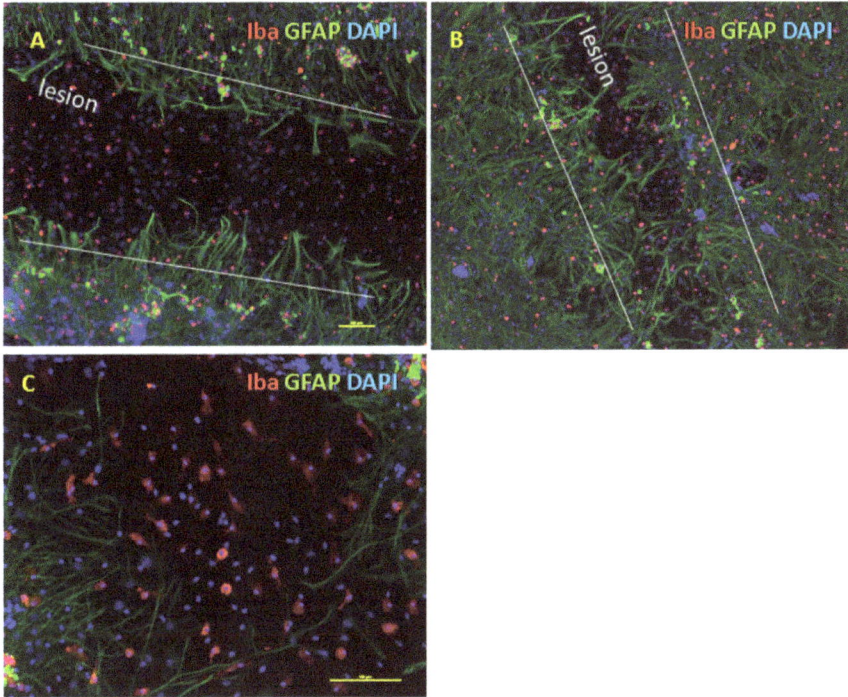

Figure 1. Fluorescent microscopy images of spinal cord culture injured by mechanical insult, control group (A) and group treated (B) with conditioned medium obtained from MSCs. The images were taken on day 2 after injury. Cells were stained with GFAP/astrocytes/green antibody, Iba/microglia cells/red antibody and DAPI/nuclear/blue marker, and (C) the detail of microglia cells infiltrating the lesion on day 2. Scale bar is 100 μm.

The cell culture approaches lack the complexity and physiological relevance of *in vivo* system. However, animal studies offer complexity, which cannot be modeled *in vitro* and which is also difficult to control and manipulate and therefore results in data that must be extrapolated to human systems [10].

3. Organotypic slices

Organotypic cultures are whole slices of tissue cultured without dissociation of the individual cells. Organotypic slices (OTSs) preserve the basic structural and connective organization of their original tissue (organotypic) and represent an interim system sharing the properties of the cell culture *in vitro* and an animal *in vivo* model. The OTS culture allows long-term maintenance of tissue architecture in "dish" [19].

OTS preparation is carried out according to the following steps. Briefly, after tissue removal under sterile conditions, the tissue is cut into 150–400 μm thick sections using a tissue chopper or vibratome. After washing, the slices are attached to a substrate and cultivated under appropriate conditions for several weeks. Today, we know many ways of OTS preparation depending on the final thickness of the slices and the survival time in culture. In *roller-tube cultures*, the slices embedded in plasma clot or collagen matrix on glass coverslips are placed in plastic culture tube containing a small amount of medium and undergo continuous slow rotation which allows the oxygenation of these slices by regular changing of the liquid–gas interface [20]. Because the slices become flattened to a quasi monolayer during cultivation procedure, this technique is appropriate when individual living nerve cells have to be observed by normal optical conditions for several weeks [21]. For obtaining quantitatively more pieces of OTSs, the modified roller method for organotypic cultivation of free-floating sections of postnatal rats can be used. This innovative procedure enables the simultaneous cultivation of multiple amount of OTS in one bottle (up to 50 and even more). For this reason, this method is advantageous for the investigation of cytotoxic injury of neural cells and appropriate immunocytochemical and molecular analysis [22]. Another, but not so frequently used, is the method, where the slices are placed either directly on collagen coated or embedded in collagen gels in Petri dishes and are totally covered by medium. These cultures survive only a few days and are mainly used for electrophysiology [21].

The most used and popular OTS-cultivating methods are the membrane cultures, where the slices are directly placed at the air–medium interface on semiporous membranes and kept stationary during the entire cultivation. Slices can collect the nutrients from an appropriate growth medium from below via capillary process and oxygen from above (**Figure 2**) [21, 23].

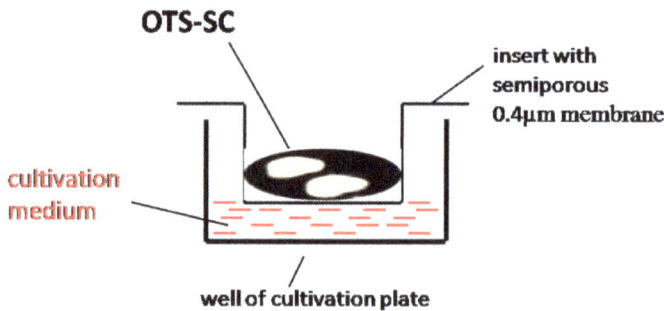

Figure 2. Schematic illustration of the most used OTS cultivating methods called "interface method". Organotypic spinal cord slice (OTS-SC) is placed on semiporous membrane through which OTS can obtain the nutrition from medium and oxygen from above.

At the beginning, experiments were carried out using hippocampal slices. However, cerebellar, cortical, and spinal cord explants have also been tested with positive results [23]. The advantage of this technique is that these OTSs are never covered with embedding materials or media which allow the study of the effect of a therapeutic agent added directly onto the OTSs during all stages of culturing longer time while maintaining semi-three-dimensional structure of tissue. Positioning of slices on the membrane is extremely easy and may represent an advantage also for co-culture experiments. This technique also has some limitations. The problem may concern the accessibility of individual neurons, because the cultured slices remain a few cell layers thick and are covered by fibers and glial processes. During OTS preparation and cultivation, we should avoid some troubles. Slices should be placed in the middle of the membrane without contacting one another. In this position, every slice can be easily reached to perform the impact injury. If any impact injury is performed, the uninjured and damaged sections have to be situated on individual insert; otherwise, excytotoxins released from damaged sections may induce injury in the controls. Sections with defective or lacking layers should be rejected from the examination. It is important to start the concrete experiments about 12–14 days after the beginning of OTS cultivation [24]. In some studies, the time of OTS culture before starting the actual experiment is shorter (1 week) [25, 26]; so the mechanical damage caused by slicing disappears, and the cells can reach a more advanced developmental stage. In addition, this time period will allow the slices to acclimatize to the culturing conditions and mature. Organotypic cultures survive from weeks to months, providing options for long-term studies, such as those studying different processes of neurodegeneration and recovery following excytotoxicity ischemia and traumatic injury.

Since the first description of organotypic hippocampal slice cultures based on the method of Gahwiler [20], the hippocampal regions are likely the most widely used organotypic slice culture model for the study of neural tissues [27]. Together with the accumulation of practical experiences and increased necessity to answer the questions dealing with nerve tissue regeneration after spinal cord injury (SCI), the development and entrenchment of organotypic spinal cord slice (OTS-SC) models became more actual. Today, there is a wide choice of methods and OTS models of both spinal cord and brain derived from different animals— mouse, rats, and rabbits [28], even the human too [29], which have been used to describe ways of monitoring spontaneous or induced neuronal degeneration in organotypic brain slice cultures [30], to study the different processes of neurodegeneration after tissue traumatic injury, and to investigate mechanisms and treatment strategies for the neurodegenerative disorders like stroke (ischemia) [31–33]. These models can simulate several pathological aspects of various neurological conditions depending on different factors, e.g., (i) the applied stimulus which causes damage, (ii) the age of OTS donor animal (iii) which parameter is the experiment focused on.

4. Insults

4.1. Ischemic insults

Damage of nerve tissue may be caused by a number of insults. Previously, organotypic slice preparations have been used in several injury models including ischemia (experimental models with oxygen-glucose deprivation) and cytotoxicity studies (exposure to glutamate receptor agonists) [24]. Ischemic insults can be generated by oxygen-glucose deprivation of the cultures by placing them for 1h in glucose-free medium saturated with 95% N_2, 5% CO_2 using standard interface method [34]. To induce stroke-like, energy failure conditions in slice cultures can be achieved in several other ways, like use of anoxic chambers or OTS submersion in glucose-free medium saturated with nitrogen [35]. In a study of free radical-induced damage in CNS using OTS exposed to H_2O_2 as a model of oxidative injury in the brain, the results provide evidence that glial cells in cultured slices are vulnerable to H_2O_2toxicity as pyramidal neurons, and that H_2O_2-mediated cell death was significantly alleviated by antioxidants and independent of calcium influx in both glial and neuronal populations [36].

The hypoxic environment in SCI has been shown to inhibit recovery. One of the promising treatments for hypoxic ischemia sustained during SCI is gene therapy. Vascular endothelial growth factor (VEGF) increasingly has gained attention as a potential factor in gene therapy to replace or improve damaged neurons in SCI because of its role in neurogenesis and neuroprotection, astrocyte proliferation, and neurite outgrowth. The controlled release of VEGF in hypoxia-inducible VEGF gene delivery system in the OTS-SC may prove to be useful for providing neuroprotection and in stimulating the neural growth in the hypoxic environment of the injured spinal cord [37]. The principal feature of acute SCI pathophysiology is excitotoxicity that is considered the main contributor to the clinical outcome. An established *in vitro* SCI model using excitotoxic damage evoked by transient kainate application to organotypic slice cultures (with predominant neuro- rather than glio-toxicity) closely mimics the *in vivo* pathophysiology of SCI. The results from such model indicate that, after an excitotoxic stimulus, extracellular S100b, a useful biomarker in serum or cerebrospinal fluid for brain or spinal cord injury, was significantly elevated in association with ongoing neuronal damage and unscathed glia [38]. The application of glutamate is believed to mimic excitotoxicity that occurs as a consequence of ischemic stroke. Also, glutamate-induced excitotoxicity is a major contributor to motor neuron (MN) degeneration in disorders such as amyotrophic lateral sclerosis, stroke, and spinal cord injury. On the basis of using OTS from different parts of SC (i.e., cervical, thoracic, and lumbar), it is found out that the MN susceptibility to glutamate-induced excitotoxicity differs within diverse populations of MNs. This sensitivity is in correlation to the segmental variable expression of glutamate receptor sub-types in MN populations. In the cervical and lumbar parts, the AMPA receptor is in dominance, whereas in thoracic segments, the NMDA receptors predominate. These results should be taken into account by devising a new drug screening experiment with cell culture system [39].

4.2. Mechanical insults

Adamchik et al. [24] described two original models of moderate mechanical trauma containing the induced primary and secondary traumatic damage in organotypic slice cultures. The primary trauma injury was achieved by quickly rolling a stainless steel cylinder (weight, 0.9 g; diameter, 5 mm; length, 7 mm) twice on the organotypic slice. To model the secondary trauma injury, a weight of 0.137 g was dropped from a height of 2 mm on a localized area of the organotypic slice. The primary damage delivered by rotating the steel cylinder on sections induces injury following the head accidents, while the damage caused in this model for secondary injury, limited initially to a small area of the section, enables to monitor the expansion of dying cells.

Almost all SCI occurring in human are due to the compression of spinal cord; therefore, most *in vitro* models have been designed to mimic this type of injury. For that reason, an *in vitro* model of neurotrauma was developed and assessed by using organotypic slice culture of adult mice spinal cord to facilitate the investigation of primary and secondary mechanisms of cell death that occur after mechanical SCI [25]. The mechanical trauma was achieved by using a weight drop model of injury, where an impactor (pin) with a weight of 0.2g was dropped from 1.7 cm onto the center of the culture slice. They modified previously described methods for generating murine spinal trauma in OTS [40]. In contrary to other models, where the OTS-SC from embryonic or neonatal mice was used, the modified model used the OTS from adult animals according to the different regenerative capabilities.

Organotypic slice cultures of spinal cord have been used in neuroscience research for a long time, but classically, these cultures were cut in the transverse plane. The transverse slices could be, however, obtained from only a single part of the spinal cord. In order to reflect the spinal cord microenvironment, the longitudinal cultures are required to maintain the basic cytoarchitectonic organization of the intact spinal cord. In contrary to the previous model, Bonnici and Kapfhammer [41] used the spinal cord slices for their study that were cut not in the transverse but in the sagittal longitudinal plane such that several spinal cord segments were included in the slide culture. This OTS-SC model is well suited for the study of axonal growth because the typical ventro-dorsal polarity of the SC is maintained after a culture period of 2 weeks, and intrinsic spinal cord axons formed a strong fiber tract extending along the longitudinal axis of the slice. The axons became myelinated during the culture period, and synaptic contacts were present in these cultures. After mechanical lesions originated by completely transecting the SC tissue with a scalpel blade, the remaining spinal cord neurons had a considerable capability to regenerate the axons. The amount of renewed axons infiltrating the wound site decreased with increasing cultivation time and maturation of the culture. This indicates that the cellular differentiation and cytoarchitectonic organization of the spinal cord neurons are similar to that of slice cultures of the transverse plane and reflects the *in vivo* situation well [41]. Some scientists use the OTS for the study of radiation effect on cell damage. By determining the time-dependent course of choline uptake in mature organotypic slice cultures of rabbit and assessing the effects of continuous and single high-dose irradiation on choline uptake, the results demonstrate that the delivery of continuous but relatively low-dose rate gamma irradiation is more efficacious than single high-dose external irradiation on high-affinity choline uptake in nervous tissues [28].

5. Age of donor animal

The age of the donor animal influences the viability of OTS, the degree of tissue organization, and the successfulness of experiment at all. Early postnatal periods (P0–P9) are ideally suited for culturing [26, 39, 42]. Since most diseases of the spinal cord concern the adults, some organotypic spinal cord slice culture models from grown rats were established [25, 26]. But the isolation of the cord from adult individuals is, however, much more problematic. The fully myelinated spinal cord is very sensitive to any damage, and cutting it with tissue chopper causes injury to about 60% of slices. The slice culture survives about 7 days maintaining proper parallel fiber tract architecture. Also, the constant high vitality and tissue organization are preserved up to 4–5 weeks in neonatal slices, while the vitality of adult slice cultures decreases significantly upon the first 5 days of cultivation [26]. On the contrary, spinal cord organotypic culture from adult mouse can be used to produce neurospheres that can be further differentiated into astrocytes and neuronal cells of different phenotypes. Although, it is not clear what exactly triggers the formation of neurospheres, one explanation could be, that neuronal loss and/or long-term culturing of spinal cord slices resets the internal cell program and stimulates proliferation and further specification of neuronal stem cells (NSCs) [43]. Most researchers did not use cultures from animals older then P6, because neuronal survival in such cultures was more variable and a longitudinal fiber tract did not develop consistently [41]. The same goes for the transverse spinal cord slice cultures, in which neuronal survival also appears to be declining in cultures derived from older postnatal animals [44].

6. Utilization of organotypic slices

Because the OTS system is accessible to experimental manipulations, OTSs represent a suitable model which may be used for different research projects not only for investigation of various parameters accompanying the CNS injury but also for the development of therapeutic application for such injury. Spinal cord injury leads to the death of various cell types, including neurons, oligodendrocytes, astrocytes, and precursor cells. A high percentage of astrocytes and oligodendrocytes in the white matter at the site of injury die within a short time after injury leading to axonal demyelination. Grafts of cells used as a treatment or as the source of supporting factors can be directly transplanted in the slices and in this way, the graft--host interaction, behavior, and fate of grafted cells can be analyzed. The injured spinal cord microenvironment is very inhospitable for survival and differentiation of transplanted or endogenous NSCs. To mimic NSC grafting into the spinal cord, NSCs were seeded on top of cultured spinal cord slices with the Hamilton syringe between 7 and 10 days after the initial culture. In such culture system, possible effects of environmental manipulation on biological behavior of either exogenous grafted NSCs or endogenous neural progenitor cells in a complex tissue environment similar to that of *in vivo* system were studied. The majority of focally applied exogenous NSCs survived up to 4 weeks, and dispersing cells did not show any preference to either the white or the gray mater. Cultured spinal cord slices retained the non-neurogenic characteristics of *in vivo* spinal cord tissue since they did not support neuronal differentiation of either exogenous NSCs or endogenous neural progenitors [42]. Also, it is very much preferred to use the OTS derived from animals with some genetic alteration, which is manifested in special disease features. For example, to study the process of the myelination and myelin support, the OTSs obtained from the cerebellum of shiverer mice were used. These mice are genetically modified in myelin basic protein (MBP) gene resulting in wide CNS dysmyelination. After the transplantation of oligodendrocyte precursors into such modified sections, the direct observation of myelin produced by grafted cells is possible. This system is more advantageous in comparison with neuron-oligodendrocyte cell co-cultures for its propinquity with *in vivo* system [45].

The impact of individual cells on the regeneration of damaged CNS tissue can be studied not only by direct transplantation of cells to OTS but also by the so-called co-culture system, where the exogenous populations are cultivated underneath the slice co-cultures without direct contact using a Transwell system. The cultured OTSs are then influenced by factors released from exogenous, co-cultured cells. Indirect co-cultivation of exogenous cells along with OTS-SC permits the analysis of the factors secreted into the medium by both cells and the spinal cord tissue and the determination of their mutual influence. For example, MSCs, the promising candidates for neuroregenerative cell therapies, promote neuronal regeneration by significantly enhanced fiber outgrowth, an effect that may be mediated by a higher expression of brain-derived neurotrophic factor (BDNF) and basic fibroblast growth factor [46]. So, the role of the MSCs is in establishing the microenvironment to be more favorable for tissue repair.

Cho et al. [47] demonstrated that the treatment of lumbar slices of spinal cord with lysolecithin caused an important degree of cell death and demyelination of nerve fibers. However, after the co-cultivation of lumbar sections with human MSCs (hMSCs), the earlier observed effects were elevated to a significant range. Since the spinal cord slice culture is totally isolated and does not have any circulating immune cells originated from the host, it excludes the possibility of any systemic immune response to transplanted human cells. The results demonstrated that direct hMSC transplantation into the demyelinated organotypic spinal cord slice culture alter the tissue microenvironment and clearly increased the survival of endogenous cells and promoted axonal outgrowth of nerves in this organotypic spinal cord slice culture. So, the OTS-SC cultures provide the opportunity to investigate the underlying mechanisms of nerve regeneration after injury in the adult nervous system and to identify the factors which enhance axonal outgrowth as well as cell survival. The ease by which organotypic slice cultures can be manipulated and inspected also make them interesting tools for studies of cell proliferation, chronic CNS astrogliosis [48] and migration [49].

The OTS could be applied also to study the neurons and glial damage during bacterial infection. In the course of pneumococcal meningitis, both spontaneous and antibiotic-induced lysis of bacteria occurs. During this process, not only cell wall constituents but also nucleic acids of the bacteria are liberated. Therefore, organotypic hippocampal slices were utilized for the investigation of possible toxic effects of complete bacteria causing meningitis or their components on neuronal and glial tissue in the absence of leukocytes. The neuronal tissue of an infected host is damaged as a result of the intense inflammatory response against the attacking bacteria. Though OTS closely mimics the *in vivo* system, during the actual cultivation, it represents only the part of more complex unit derived from, which is closed without any circulating immune cells. According to this, by the measurement of neuron-specific enolase in cultivation medium, as an additional indicator of neuronal damage, it was found out that not only heat-inactivated whole bacteria but also diverse bacterial elements were capable of inducing nervous tissue damage, such as bacterial walls and nucleic acids [50]. Also, the organotypic brain slice cultures of bovine origin are a suitable model to study aspects of host–pathogen interaction in listeric encephalitis and potentially in other neuroinfectious diseases [51]. To evaluate the effect of HIV-1 virus on neural cells, a method for culturing human fetal organotypic brain slices in the presence of live virus was developed. The brain--derived OTSs were maintained on membranes, and co-cultured with HIV-1–infected T-cells on the well bottom. Thus, OTSs were exposed to live virus during whole cultivation time, HIV-1 proteins, and other molecules produced by the infected T-cells. The results obtained from this model indicate the gliosis observed *in vivo*. This valuable method can be used to model the dynamics and the microenvironment of brain tissue exposed to HIV-1 and can eventually be used to test therapies directed at preventing HIV-1-induced neural damage in CNS [52].

Within the wide range of available OTSs derived from different CNS sections, the OTS-SC system represents an attractive model with some benefits, when compared to generally used *in vitro* and *in vivo* models. OTS-SC can be kept under cultivation conditions for a long time. During the whole cultivation time, this system enables quick and direct evaluation and identification of huge diapason of different cellular, molecular relations involved in regeneration processes. Moreover, OTS-SCs can be utilized to improve the *ex vivo* neurological disorders and thus represent an intermediate step between *in vitro* experiments and animal models [53].

7. Experimental study

The aim of our study was: (i) to imitate the spinal cord injury (SCI) in organotypic spinal cord slice (OTS-SC) and (ii) to treat these injured OTS-SCs (OTS-SCIs) in the presence of rat mesenchymal stem cells (rMSCs). We imitate the SCI in the OTS-SC not by direct mechanical impact, but the injury was induced by OTS-SC treated with conditioned medium obtained from injured spinal cord (CM-SCI). CM-SCI represents a cocktail of cytokines and chemokines released by central lesion segments of injured spinal cord. We examined the impact of CM-SCI, as well as rMSCs on behavior of microglia cells, astrocytes, and neurons in the organotypic spinal cord slice cultures.

7.1. Methods

The SCI was induced by modified balloon-compression technique in adult rats [54], and after 3 days of animal survival, the central lesion segments were dissected and cultured for 24 h *in vitro* to obtain CM-SCI used for OTS-SC treatment. Similarly, we obtained the conditioned medium from control-intact thoracic spinal cord (CM-SC), which in our experiment served as a source of control-conditioned medium. The OTS-SCs were prepared from lumbar SCs of naive adult male rats. The isolated SCs were transversely cut with a McIlwain tissue chopper into 400 μm OTS-SC sections and cultivated for an adaptation for 5 days in 1ml/well of culture media containing DMEM, 10% fetal bovine serum, and 1% penicillin–streptomycin and incubated at 37°C in humidified atmosphere with 5% of CO_2 using standard interface method. The study was performed with the approval and guidelines of the Institutional Animal Care and Use Committee of the Slovak Academy of Sciences and with the European Communities Council Directive (2010/63/EU) regarding the use of animals in Research, Slovak Law for Animal Protection No. 377/2012 and 436/2012.

7.2. *In vitro* model of spinal cord injury and treatment

After adaptation, OTS-SCs were divided into four groups according to the treatment and cultivated for the next 3 days. (i) **OTS-SC** (OTS treated with CM-SC), (ii) **OTS-SCI** (OTS treated with CM-SCI) (iii) **OTS-SC + MSCs** (OTS co-cultured with rMSCs in CM-SC), and (iv) **OTS-SCI + MSCs** (OTS co-cultured with rMSCs in CM-SCI) (**Figure 3**).

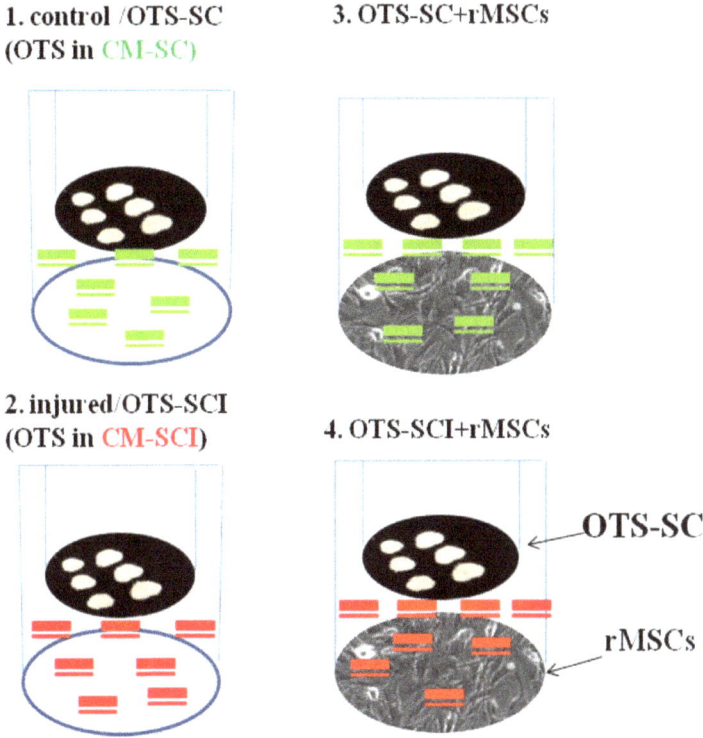

Figure 3. The design of the experiment. After adaptation, OTS-SCs were divided into four groups according to the treatment and cultivated for the next three days. Control group is represented by OTS-SCs treated with conditioned medium obtained from intact spinal cord. OTS-SCs treated with conditioned medium from injured spinal cord represent *in vitro* model of spinal cord injury. Both groups were co-cultured with mesenchymal stem cells to investigate the potential influence of these cells on behavior of different cell population in OTSs.

Rat MSCs were isolated from bone marrow of the long bones (femur, tibia) of adult male Wistar rats (290–320 g). To confirm the phenotypic characteristics of rMSC of the third passage, the surface markers (CD29, CD90, and CD45) were analyzed by flow cytometry [55]. The co-culture of rMSCs with OTS-SCs started at the same time with CM-SCI or CM-SC influence. On the basis of immunohistochemistry analyses for cell markers (Iba-microglial cells, GFAP-astrocytes, NeuN-neurons), after 3 days of treatment, OTS-SCs were analyzed using a Leica SP5X confocal microscope and an inverted Nikon ECLIPSE Ti fluorescence microscope. We examined the percentage of NeuN and Iba positive cells calculated from the total number of DAPI (4′,6-diamidino-2-phenylindole) - positive cells in 10 random visual fields (600 × 600 μm) in OTSs. The quantification of immunofluorescence intensity of GFAP positive cells was also analyzed by Image J software according to the previous protocol [56]. Data are presented as mean ± SEM. Statistical differences between groups were evaluated with ANOVA, and values of *$p < 0.05$ and **$p < 0.01$ were considered to be statistically significant.

7.3. Results

During the cultivation time, slices preserved their morphological and structural integrity with clear differentiation of white and gray matter. In response to injury induced by conditioned medium from injured spinal cord, both astrocytes and microglia were activated, while astrocytes served as a stimulus for microglial-mediated inflammation.

The highest positivity of the microglial populations was observed in the injured OTS-SCI group $(3.98 \pm 0.64\%)$ when compared to control OTS-SC $(1.36 \pm 0.46\%, **p < 0.01)$ and OTS-SC + MSCs $(1.22 \pm 0.62\%, **p < 0.01)$ (**Figure 4**). OTS-SCI represents *in vitro* model of spinal cord injury. The treatment in *in vitro* model of spinal cord injury with MSCs, in OTS-SCI + MSCs group, caused a significant decrease of microglial cell population $(2.9 \pm 0.85\%, *p < 0.05)$ in comparison with the actual *in vitro* model of spinal cord injury. Astrocytes showed a similar pattern of behavior like microglia cells. The highest activation of astrocytes was observed in the OTS-SCI $(density/25.26 \pm 3.29)$ in comparison with the OTS-SC $(density/14.31 \pm 4.33, *p < 0.05)$ and OTS-SCI + MSCs $(density/19.52 \pm 5.22, *p < 0.05)$ groups (**Figure 5**). We observed an adverse impact of CM-SCI on the neuron presence in slices. The smallest number of the neurons $(4.38 \pm 1.77\%)$ was found in the injured OTS-SCI slices. The co-culture with MSCs elevated the amount of the neurons $(13.78 \pm 4.51\%, **p < 0.01)$ in OTS-SC + MSCs when compared to actual *in vitro* model (**Figure 6**).

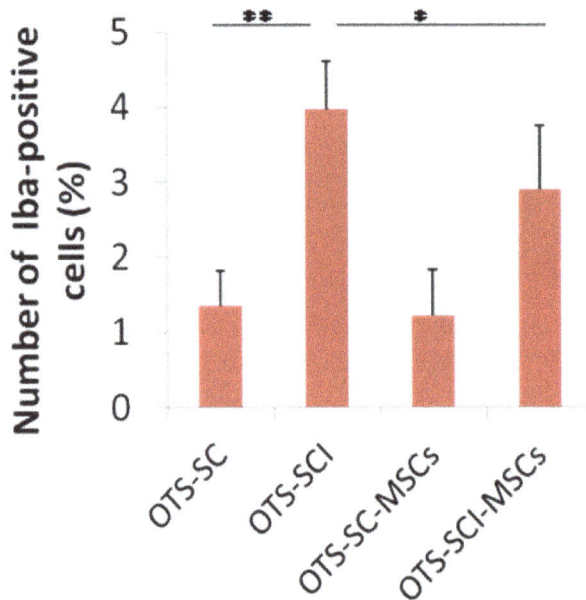

Figure 4. The number of Iba positive microglia cells observed in OTS-SCs treated with conditioned medium from intact/injured spinal cord OTS-SC/OTS-SCI and co-cultured with mesenchymal stem cells. Cultivation of spinal cord slices in CM-SCI caused a significant increase in number of microglial positive cells when compared to controls. Besides, co-cultivation of injured OTS with MSCs (OTS-SCI + MSCs) inhibits the activation of microglial cells causing a significant decrease of Iba positive cells in comparison to untreated *in vitro* model of spinal cord injury (OTS-SCI).

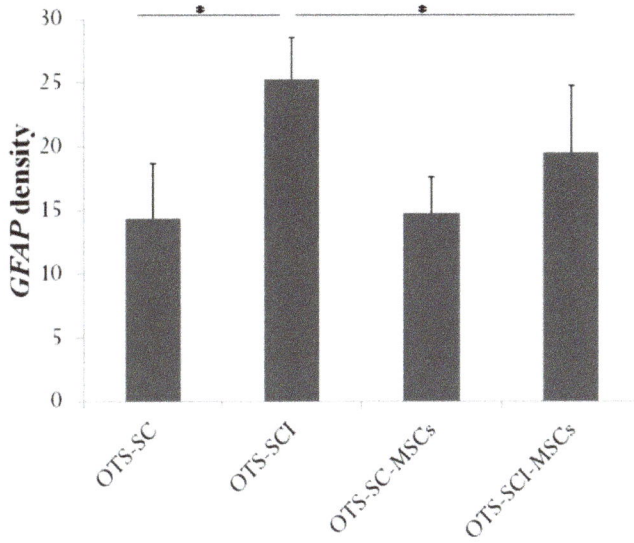

Figure 5. The GFAP density detected in OTS-SCs treated with conditioned medium from intact/injured spinal cord OTS-SC/OTS-SCI and co-cultured with mesenchymal stem cells. The highest activation of astrocytes was observed in the OTS-SCI and co-cultivation of injured OTS with MSCs (OTS-SCI + MSCs) caused a significant decrease of astrocytes when compared to untreated *in vitro* model of spinal cord injury (OTS-SCI).

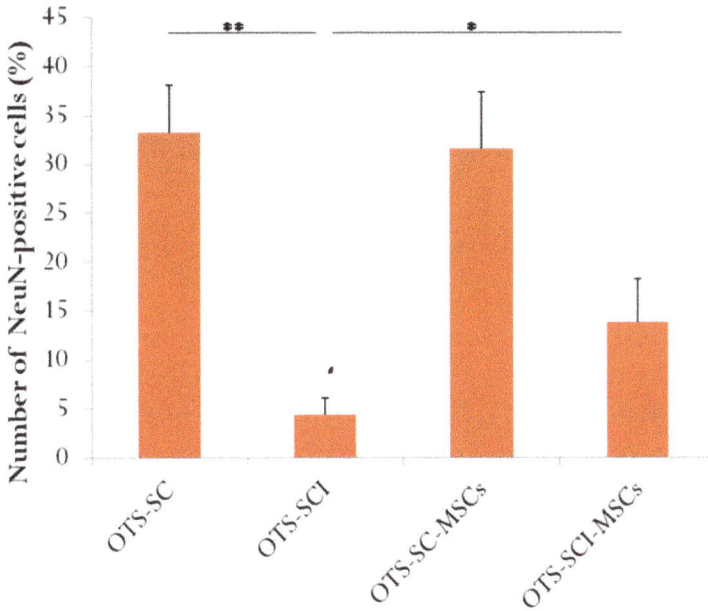

Figure 6. The number of NeuN positive cells noted in spinal cord slices treated with conditioned medium from intact/injured spinal cord OTS-SC/OTS-SCI and co-cultured with mesenchymal stem cells. Cultivation of spinal cord slices in CM-SCI caused a significant decrease in number of neuronal cells when compared to controls. MSCs have neurotrophic effects resulting in an increase of neuronal cells in *in vitro* model of spinal cord injury treated with MSCs (OTS-SCI + MSCs).

Our data revealed increased activity of microglia and astrocytes and elimination of neurons in experimental group treated with CM-SCI. We observed the presence of hypertrophied astrocytes with increased proliferation activity within the white matter of injured experimental group in contrary to controls. Astrocytes are one of the major glial cell types that maintain homeostasis in the undamaged CNS. After injury, astrocytes become reactive and prevent regeneration; however, it has also been suggested that astrocytes can become activated and promote regeneration. This indicated that reactive astrogliosis may exert both beneficial and detrimental effects in a context-specific manner determined by distinct molecular signaling cascades. Resident microglia in the control group OTS-SC was in the resting state and cells were few in number and smaller in size (**Figure 7A**). After inducing damage effects in the OTS-SCI with CM-SCI, quiescent microglial cells became activated, were bigger, and created ramified processes (**Figure 7B**).

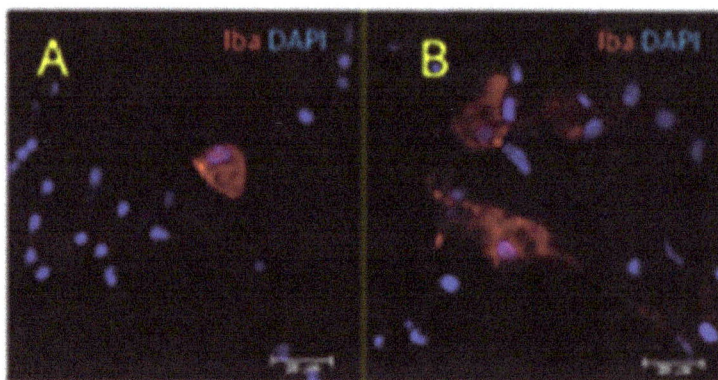

Figure 7. Fluorescent microscopy images of the residual microglia (red) in organotypic spinal cord slices (400 μm) stained with specific Iba antibody. The immunoreactive cells in control OTS-SC group (A) and injured OTS-SCI group (B). Scale bar is 10 μm.

Our study showed that (i) OTS-SC *in vitro* model closely mimics the post-injury microenvironment affecting the microglia and astrocytes cell response following secondary damage and is suitable for various pharmacy-therapeutic approaches, and that (ii) rMSCs are able to inhibit the activation of microglial cells and have neurotrophic effects on the neural cells. Thus, the effects shown in this study are directly mediated from various factors or proteins secreted from rMSCs. Our study represents the rMSC as a promising candidate for SCI treatment due to their potential to perform the immunomodulatory functions and to produce specific neurotrophic components and cytokines likewise to other results [57]. These techniques give us the possibility to achieve a moderate trauma in *in vitro* preparation, the organotypic slices that can be used to study short- and long-term effects and mechanisms of traumatic injury. Our study supports the recent hypothesis regarding the role of MSCs in establishing microenvironment more favorable for tissue repair. MSCs have a great potential in therapy for a range of neural insults.

8. Summary

Many *in vitro* models are invented, and others are still waiting for their further application, depending on the interest of researchers and key problems they are focused on. Many *in vitro* models are used in bright research field concerning the influence of any factor originated due to human activity we come into contact every day. For example, exposure of primary rat cortical neurons to extremely low-frequency electromagnetic fields has only limited (developmental) neurotoxic potential *in vitro* manifested by unchanged cell viability and neurite outgrowth [58]. Organotypic slice cultures have the potential to become powerful tools in the arsenal of drug discovery technology, lying at the interface between high-throughput screening and clinically relevant animal disease models. It has to be mentioned, however, that the cultured slices cannot represent all the *in vivo* properties. However, organotypic slices can model different histopathological aspects of neurological conditions and are a suitable *in vitro* system to address a wide range of questions concerning mechanisms of nerve regeneration after injury in the adult nervous system and to identify the factors supporting or preventing axonal outgrowth as well as cell survival that will ultimately add to the development of therapeutic application for spinal cord injury. Organotypic culture technique is easy, efficient, and practical and allows reduction of animal number and preserves the three-dimensional neuronal network. Although these *in vitro* organotypic slices have been able to model and reproduce many processes taking place after CNS injury with subsequent regeneration, some limitations exist, including the lack of any functioning vasculature, an incomplete immune system. Thus, OTSs have their own advantages and disadvantages with regard to stimulating *in vivo* conditions. Obviously, organotypic slices cannot replace *in vivo* models, which are still necessary and remain the only way to evaluate the functional outcome of a therapeutic strategy [59].

Acknowledgements

We acknowledge the financial support given by the Grant Agency of the Slovak Academy of Sciences: VEGA 2/0169/13, VEGA 2/0125/15, and VEGA 2/0145/16.

Author details

Lucia Slovinska*, Juraj Blasko, Miriam Nagyova, Eva Szekiova and Dasa Cizkova

*Address all correspondence to: slovinska@saske.sk

Institute of Neurobiology, Slovak Academy of Sciences, Kosice, Slovakia

References

[1] Rowland J, Hawryluk GW, Kwon B, Fehlings MG: Current status of acute spinal cord injury pathophysiology and emerging therapies: promise on the horizon. Neurosurg Focus 2008; 25: E2.

[2] Fawcett JW, Asher RA: The glial scar and central nervous system repair. Brain Res Bull 1999; 49: 377–391.

[3] Rudge JS, Silver J: Inhibition of neurite outgrowth on astroglial scars in vitro. J Neurosci 1990; 10: 3594–3603.

[4] Tom VJ, Steinmetz MP, Miller JH, Doller CM, Silver J: Studies on the development and behavior of the dystrophic growth cone, the hallmark of regeneration failure, in an in vitro model of the glial scar and after spinal cord injury. J Neurosci 2004; 24: 6531–6539.

[5] Boomkamp SD, McGrath MA, Houslay MD, Barnett SC: Epac and the high affinity rolipram binding conformer of PDE4 modulate neurite outgrowth and myelination using an in vitro spinal cord injury model. Br J Pharmacol 2014; 171: 2385–2398.

[6] Slovinska L, Szekiova E, Blasko J, Devaux S, Salzet M, Cizkova D: Comparison of dynamic behavior and maturation of neural multipotent cells derived from different spinal cord developmental stages: an in vitro study. Acta Neurobiol Exp (Wars) 2015; 75: 107–114.

[7] Morrison B, 3rd, Saatman KE, Meaney DF, McIntosh TK: In vitro central nervous system models of mechanically induced trauma: a review. J Neurotrauma 1998; 15: 911–928.

[8] Shearer MC, Niclou SP, Brown D, Asher RA, Holtmaat AJ, Levine JM, Verhaagen J, Fawcett JW: The astrocyte/meningeal cell interface is a barrier to neurite outgrowth which can be overcome by manipulation of inhibitory molecules or axonal signalling pathways. Mol Cell Neurosci 2003; 24: 913–925.

[9] Wanner IB, Deik A, Torres M, Rosendahl A, Neary JT, Lemmon VP, Bixby JL: A new in vitro model of the glial scar inhibits axon growth. Glia 2008; 56: 1691–1709.

[10] Hopkins AM, DeSimone E, Chwalek K, Kaplan DL: 3D in vitro modeling of the central nervous system. Prog Neurobiol 2015; 125: 1–25.

[11] Boomkamp SD, Riehle MO, Wood J, Olson MF, Barnett SC: The development of a rat in vitro model of spinal cord injury demonstrating the additive effects of Rho and ROCK inhibitors on neurite outgrowth and myelination. Glia 2012; 60: 441–456.

[12] Kim BG, Hwang DH, Lee SI, Kim EJ, Kim SU: Stem cell-based cell therapy for spinal cord injury. Cell Transplant 2007; 16: 355–364.

[13] Nash B, Thomson CE, Linington C, Arthur AT, McClure JD, McBride MW, Barnett SC: Functional duality of astrocytes in myelination. J Neurosci 2011; 31: 13028–13038.

[14] Ioannidou K, Edgar JM, Barnett SC: Time-lapse imaging of glial-axonal interactions. Curr Protoc Neurosci 2012; 72: 2.23.21–22.23.14.

[15] Ioannidou K, Anderson KI, Strachan D, Edgar JM, Barnett SC: Astroglial–axonal interactions during early stages of myelination in mixed cultures using in vitro and ex vivo imaging techniques. BMC Neurosci 2014; 15: 59.

[16] Sorensen A, Moffat K, Thomson C, Barnett SC: Astrocytes, but not olfactory ensheathing cells or Schwann cells, promote myelination of CNS axons in vitro. Glia 2008; 56: 750–763.

[17] Al-Ali H, Beckerman S, Bixby JL, Lemmon VP: In vitro models of axon regeneration. Exp Neurol 2016. In press - doi:10.1016/j.expneurol.2016.01.020

[18] Ribeiro C, Slgado AJ, Fraga JS, Silva NA, Reis RL, Sousa N: The secretome of bone marrow mesenchymal stem cells-conditioned media varies with time and drives a distinct effect on mature neurons and glial cells (primary cultures). J Tissue Eng Regen Med 2011; DOI: 10.1002/term.

[19] Gahwiler BH: Organotypic cultures of neural tissue. Trends Neurosci 1988; 11: 484–489.

[20] Gahwiler BH: Organotypic monolayer cultures of nervous tissue. J Neurosci Methods 1981; 4: 329–342.

[21] Gahwiler BH, Capogna M, Debanne D, McKinney RA, Thompson SM: Organotypic slice cultures: a technique has come of age. Trends Neurosci 1997; 20: 471–477.

[22] Victorov IV, Lyjin AA, Aleksandrova OP: A modified roller method for organotypic brain cultures: free-floating slices of postnatal rat hippocampus. Brain Res Protoc 2001; 7: 30–37.

[23] Stoppini L, Buchs PA, Muller D: A simple method for organotypic cultures of nervous tissue. J Neurosci Methods 1991; 37: 173–182.

[24] Adamchik Y, Frantseva MV, Weisspapir M, Carlen PL, Perez Velazquez JL: Methods to induce primary and secondary traumatic damage in organotypic hippocampal slice cultures. Brain Res Protoc 2000; 5: 153–158.

[25] Krassioukov AV, Ackery A, Schwartz G, Adamchik Y, Liu Y, Fehlings MG: An in vitro model of neurotrauma in organotypic spinal cord cultures from adult mice. Brain Res Protoc 2002; 10: 60–68.

[26] Sypecka J, Koniusz S, Kawalec M, Sarnowska A: The organotypic longitudinal spinal cord slice culture for stem cell study. Stem Cells Int 2015; 2015: 471216.

[27] Förster E, Bartos M, Zhao S: Hippocampal slice cultures. In: Poindron P, Piguet P, Förster E (eds.) New methods for culturing cells from nervous tissues. BioValley Monogr, vol. 1. Basel, Karger; 2005: p. 1–11.

[28] Savas A, Warnke PC, Ginap T, Feuerstein TJ, Ostertag CB: The effects of continuous and single-dose radiation on choline uptake in organotypic tissue slice cultures of rabbit hippocampus. Neurol Res 2001; 23: 669–675.

[29] Jeong D, Taghavi CE, Song KJ, Lee KB, Kang HW: Organotypic human spinal cord slice culture as an alternative to direct transplantation of human bone marrow precursor cells for treating spinal cord injury. World Neurosurg 2011; 75: 533–539.

[30] Noraberg J, Kristensen BW, Zimmer J: Markers for neuronal degeneration in organotypic slice cultures. Brain Res Protoc 1999; 3: 278–290.

[31] Morrison B, 3rd, Eberwine JH, Meaney DF, McIntosh TK: Traumatic injury induces differential expression of cell death genes in organotypic brain slice cultures determined by complementary DNA array hybridization. Neuroscience 2000; 96: 131–139.

[32] Ravikumar M, Jain S, Miller RH, Capadona JR, Selkirk SM: An organotypic spinal cord slice culture model to quantify neurodegeneration. J Neurosci Methods 2012; 211: 280–288.

[33] Noraberg J, Poulsen FR, Blaabjerg M, Kristensen BW, Bonde C, Montero M, Meyer M, Gramsbergen JB, Zimmer J: Organotypic hippocampal slice cultures for studies of brain damage, neuroprotection and neurorepair. Curr Drug Targets CNS Neurol Disord 2005; 4: 435–452.

[34] Sundstrom L, Morrison B, 3rd, Bradley M, Pringle A: Organotypic cultures as tools for functional screening in the CNS. Drug Discov Today 2005; 10: 993–1000.

[35] Frantseva MV, Carlen PL, El-Beheiry H: A submersion method to induce hypoxic damage in organotypic hippocampal cultures. J Neurosci Methods 1999; 89: 25–31.

[36] Feeney CJ, Frantseva MV, Carlen PL, Pennefather PS, Shulyakova N, Shniffer C, Mills LR: Vulnerability of glial cells to hydrogen peroxide in cultured hippocampal slices. Brain Res 2008; 1198: 1–15.

[37] An SS, Pennant WA, Ha Y, Oh JS, Kim HJ, Gwak SJ, Yoon DH, Kim KN: Hypoxia-induced expression of VEGF in the organotypic spinal cord slice culture. Neuroreport 2011; 22: 55–60.

[38] Mazzone GL, Nistri A: S100beta as an early biomarker of excitotoxic damage in spinal cord organotypic cultures. J Neurochem 2014; 130: 598–604.

[39] Nava J, Mayorenko II, Grehl T, Steinbuch HWM, Weis J, Brook GA: Differential pattern of neuroprotection in lumbar, cervical and thoracic spinal cord segments in an organotypic rat model of glutamate-induced excitotoxicity. J Chem Neuroanat 2013; 53: 11–17.

[40] Balentine JD, Greene WB, Bornstein M: In vitro spinal cord trauma. Lab Invest 1988; 58: 93–99.

[41] Bonnici B, Kapfhammer JP: Spontaneous regeneration of intrinsic spinal cord axons in a novel spinal cord slice culture model. Eur J Neurosci 2008; 27: 2483–2492.

[42] Kim HM, Lee HJ, Lee MY, Kim SU, Kim BG: Organotypic spinal cord slice culture to study neural stem/progenitor cell microenvironment in the injured spinal cord. Exp Neurobiol 2010; 19: 106–113.

[43] Glazova MV, Pak ES, Murashov AK: Neurogenic potential of spinal cord organotypic culture. Neurosci Lett 2015; 594: 60–65.

[44] Delfs J, Friend J, Ishimoto S, Saroff D: Ventral and dorsal horn acetylcholinesterase neurons are maintained in organotypic cultures of postnatal rat spinal cord explants. Brain Res 1989; 488: 31–42.

[45] Bin JM, Leong SY, Bull SJ, Antel JP, Kennedy TE: Oligodendrocyte precursor cell transplantation into organotypic cerebellar shiverer slices: a model to study myelination and myelin maintenance. PLoS One 2012; 7: e41237.

[46] Sygnecka K, Heider A, Scherf N, Alt R, Franke H, Heine C: Mesenchymal stem cells support neuronal fiber growth in an organotypic brain slice co-culture model. Stem Cells Dev 2014; 24: 824–835.

[47] Cho JS, Park HW, Park SK, Roh S, Kang SK, Paik KS, Chang MS: Transplantation of mesenchymal stem cells enhances axonal outgrowth and cell survival in an organotypic spinal cord slice culture. Neurosci Lett 2009; 454: 43–48.

[48] Dean JM, Riddle A, Maire J, Hansen KD, Preston M, Barnes AP, Sherman LS, Back SA: An organotypic slice culture model of chronic white matter injury with maturation arrest of oligodendrocyte progenitors. Mol Neurodegener 2011; 6: 46.

[49] Ngalula KP, Cramer N, Schell MJ, Juliano SL: Transplanted neural progenitor cells from distinct sources migrate differentially in an organotypic model of brain injury. Front Neurol 2015; 6: 212.

[50] Schmidt H, Tlustochowska A, Stuertz K, Djukic M, Gerber J, Schutz E, Kuhnt U, Nau R: Organotypic hippocampal cultures. A model of brain tissue damage in Streptococcus pneumoniae meningitis. J Neuroimmunol 2001; 113: 30–39.

[51] Guldimann C, Lejeune B, Hofer S, Leib SL, Frey J, Zurbriggen A, Seuberlich T, Oevermann A: Ruminant organotypic brain-slice cultures as a model for the investigation of CNS listeriosis. Int J Exp Pathol 2012; 93: 259–268.

[52] Martinez R, Eraso D, Geffin R, McCarthy M: A two-culture method for exposure of human brain organotypic slice cultures to replicating human immunodeficiency virus type 1. J Neurosci Methods 2011; 200: 74–79.

[53] Pandamooz S, Nabiuni M, Miyan J, Ahmadiani A, Dargahi L: Organotypic spinal cord culture: a proper platform for the functional screening. Mol Neurobiol 2015. DOI 10.1007/s12035-015-9403-z

[54] Vanicky I, Urdzikova L, Saganova K, Cizkova D, Galik J: A simple and reproducible model of spinal cord injury induced by epidural balloon inflation in the rat. J Neurotrauma 2001; 18: 1399–1407.

[55] Nagyova M, Slovinska L, Blasko J, Grulova I, Kuricova M, Cigankova V, Harvanova D, Cizkova D: A comparative study of PKH67, DiI, and BrdU labeling techniques for tracing rat mesenchymal stem cells. In Vitro Cell Dev Biol Anim 2014; 50: 656–663.

[56] Jones LL, Tuszynski MH: Spinal cord injury elicits expression of keratan sulfate proteoglycans by macrophages, reactive microglia, and oligodendrocyte progenitors. J Neurosci 2002; 22: 4611–4624.

[57] Bai L, Lennon DP, Caplan AI, DeChant A, Hecker J, Kranso J, Zaremba A, Miller R: Hepatocyte growth factor mediates MSCs stimulated functional recovery in animal models of MS. Nat Neurosci 2012; 15: 862–870.

[58] de Groot MW, van Kleef RG, de Groot A, Westerink RH: In vitro developmental neurotoxicity following chronic exposure to 50 Hz extremely low-frequency electromagnetic fields in primary rat cortical cultures. Toxicol Sci 2016; 149: 433–440.

[59] Daviaud N, Garbayo E, Schiller PC, Perez-Pinzon M, Montero-Menei CN: Organotypic cultures as tools for optimizing central nervous system cell therapies. Exp Neurol 2013; 248: 429–440.

7

Orthoses for Spinal Cord Injury Patients

Mokhtar Arazpour, Monireh Ahmadi Bani,
Mohammad Ebrahim Mousavi,
Mahmood Bahramizadeh and
Mohammad Ali Mardani

Abstract

There are some limitations for patients with spinal cord injury (SCI) when walking with assistive devices. Heavy energy expenditure and walking high loads on the upper limb joints are two main reasons of high rejection rate of orthosis by these patients . Many devices have been designed to enable people with paraplegia to ambulate in an upright position as a solution of these limitations such as mechanical orthoses, hybrid orthoses and powered orthoses. All these devices are designed to solve the problem of standing and walking, but there are some other important notes, which should be considered. For example, the size and weight of external orthoses, donning and doffing, cumbersomeness and independency for using are very important.

Keywords: spinal cord injury, orthoses, walking, assistive devices

1. Introduction

Lower limb paralysis resulting from spinal cord injury (SCI) causes inability to walk. Trauma is one of the main causes of SCI that occurs mostly in young people (aged between 16 and 30 years). In 2006, more than 2000 patients with SCI were in the United States and there are more than 10,000 new cases each year [1]. The ability to walk is the ultimate goal of rehabilitation in SCI patients. Ambulation is always influenced in patients with SCI based on the lesion level and the resulting different levels of muscle paralysis, sensory impairment, spasticity and the lack of trunk control. Walking anomalies in patients with SCI included the absence of active sagittal plane motions in the hip and knee joints, increased ankle plantarflexion during swing phase and an inability to positioning the lower extremity for initial foot contact and the existence of the so-called "foot slap" based on paralysis of ankle dorsiflexor muscles. Different types of orthoses are designed to reduce complication of inability to walk.

In this chapter, we introduce different types of orthoses for patients with spinal cord injury and explain important parameters (walking, stability, energy expenditure and independency) for all existent orthoses by current documents.

2. Different types of orthoses

In overall view, there were three mechanisms in orthoses to walking in spinal cord injury patients: mechanical orthoses, hybrid orthoses and power orthoses (exoskeleton).

2.1. Mechanical orthoses

In this category, three types of the mechanical orthoses included were hip-knee-ankle-foot orthoses, reciprocating gait orthoses and medial linkage orthoses.

2.1.1. Hip-knee-ankle-foot orthoses

A simple hip joint with one degree of freedom generally was used in the Hip Knee Ankle Foot Orthosis (HKAFO). Paraplegic patients use a swing through walking pattern during ambulation with this type of orthoses. Walking with this pattern produces a high rate of energy consumption and high rate of loads on the upper limb joints (shoulder joints and wrist) in paraplegic patients [2–5].

2.1.2. Reciprocating gait orthoses

Reciprocating gait orthoses (RGO) were introduced in the late 1960s. The ultimate goal was mobilizing lower limb by trunk extension. Therefore, hip extension in one side created hip flexion in other side. In using this kind of orthosis, patients were able to walk reciprocally, doff and don the orthosis independently, but cannot stand up without assistance [6, 7]. In addition, walking on a ramp and incline is difficult for paraplegic patients when using the original form of RGO [6]. To resolve this problem, the hip joints in this orthosis must have a two condition locking systems: firstly, in a full extension locking position and secondly in 20° flexion from the first position to walking on ramp and incline [6].

A modified version of RGOs is referred to as the Advanced Reciprocating Gait Orthosis (ARGO) with a one pull-push cable within the pelvic section developed to assist walking performance in paraplegic subjects. In comparison, the Hip Guidance Orthosis (HGO), RGO and ARGO demonstrated the same motion in pattern and magnitude, but in using the ARGO the pelvic displayed a jerky movement pattern. A more developed RGO is defined as the Isocentric Reciprocating Gait Orthosis (IRGO) and was introduced by Motlock in 1992 [8].

2.1.3. *Medial linkage orthosis (MLO)*

Another type of mechanical orthosis is medial linkage orthosis (MLO). There are variations in this type of orthosis, which include the WalkAbout (WA) [9], Moorong [10] and PrimeWalk (PW) [11] and the Hip and Ankle Linked Orthosis (HALO) [12]. These orthosis are based on a medial single hip joint, which provides artificial hip joint movements. Although it is noted that there is no congruency between the anatomical and mechanical hip joints in the Walkabout MLO, this limitation has been resolved in the Primewalk and Moorong MLO [9–11].

Evaluation of the hip joint mechanism when using the IRGO has been reported to demonstrate improved gait parameters, energy consumption compared to other RGOs, HKAFO and MLOs [13]. Therefore, the prescribed option in improvement of walking parameters between mechanical orthoses is the IRGO system. The difference between walking with optimal mechanical orthoses (IRGO) and healthy subjects walking is high. Donning and doffing with this type of orthosis, however, is difficult due to its bulky structure and increased weight. MLOs have less donning and doffing time and light structure compared to IRGOs, but these types of orthoses do not have a reciprocating gait mechanism and pelvic rigid structure. Therefore, the users are forced to use high energy consumption during walking, which in turn can create a poor posture compared to walking with IRGO conditions [13–15].

Walking with a mechanical orthoses is not ideal for SCI patients and is a view based on the associated problems during walking with them that includes high loads on upper limb joints and high rate of energy consumption. Some authors have also stated that walking with mechanical orthoses is boring and exhausted [2, 4, 7, 16]. Recent efforts to improve orthoses for SCI patients have led to systems of orthoses that combine the mechanical orthoses with functional electrical stimulation of selected lower extremity muscles and powered hip orthoses [3, 17–19]. Generally, walking parameters and energy consumption improved with new generation of orthoses [19, 20].

2.2. Hybrid orthoses

Hybrid orthoses are a kind of orthoses, which are activated by functional electrical stimulation (FES). FES is the application of external electrical stimulation to paralyzed muscles to restore their function [6]. The first reported use of FES to facilitate walking for SCI individuals was in 1980, involving the stimulation of quadriceps muscle to enhance stability during stance phase. Two kinds of hybrid orthoses are available: hybrid orthosis based on available mechanical designs (HGO, LSU RGO, ARGO and MLO) and hybrid orthoses based on the new designs (modular hybrid, wrapped spring clutch and spring brake orthoses).

Although some benefits are noted about hybrid orthosis, there are some limitation associated with the use of orthoses, FES or hybrid orthoses, which include premature muscle fatigue, false triggering of nearby muscles and being heavy and orthotics cumbersomeness.

2.3. Power orthoses (exoskeleton)

Powered orthoses (exoskeleton) are kinds of orthoses, which activate with external power. The mechanical orthoses have a simple structure and user-friendly design. This type of orthoses, however, has not progressed in development in recent years with the progression, since technology of the powered orthoses appears to be the main focus of research in rehabilitation and assisted walking and ambulation in SCI patients. There is currently only a limited range of powered orthoses, but there is some evidence of an increase in temporal spatial parameters when walking with powered orthoses [21, 22].

One successful approach used in patient rehabilitation is the use of partial weight bearing when walking on a treadmill using suspension via an overhead harness. This technique, known as body weight support treadmill training (BWSTT), has been used to encourage the regeneration of stepping and walking in incomplete and complete SCI subjects [23, 24]. One of the limitations of BWSTT is that it can only be used in a clinical environment. Provision of hip extension at the end of stance phase, adequate weight bearing through the lower limb during stance phase and the ability to shift weight to the lateral side in the double support phase are essential for BWSTT [25]. However, agreement on the ideal parameters of such gait training does not currently exist [26]. The speed of the treadmill [27], cadence used, and the amount of body unloading are parameters, which can affect gait training in SCI subjects using this system [28]. Therefore, due to these limitations, powered gait orthosis (PGOs) may offer potential in providing an alternative form of gait training for SCI patients.

PGOs can be used as a gait training system to facilitate ambulation in both the clinical situation and in the home via an external power supply using electric motors, pneumatic and/or hydraulic actuators [9]. The first design and construction of PGOs were done in mid-1970s [29]. Belforte [30, 31], and Kang et al. [32], both developed powered orthoses with pneumatic actuators, which demonstrated a positive effect on walking by paraplegic patients, and further developments were subsequently reported by Ruthenberg et al. [33], Ohta et al. [34] and Arazpour et al. [35, 36].

Robert Bogue analyzed some recently developed exoskeletons for military, civil and medical applications and described brain-computer and systems in this review paper [37]. Ferris et al. in another review paper evaluated the recent powered lower limb orthosis for assisting treadmill stepping in disable persons. Practice starting, turning, stopping and avoiding obstacles during overground walking reported main advantage of using powered orthoses as rehabilitation aids in gait rehabilitation after neurological injury. In this study, the powered orthosis that used with bodyweight supported treadmill training for gait rehabilitation in clinical environment analyzed [38]. In the review paper, Dollar and Herr reported the history of the lower limb active orthoses. They reported a design overview of hardware, actuation, sensory and control systems for most of the powered orthosis that have been fabricated until 2007 [39]. Powered orthosis in this literature included full lower limb exoskeletons, modular active orthoses, single joint active orthoses and other orthotic devices. They conducted that the research directions in the future will focus more on the development of light weight exoskeletons and active orthotic devices. All powered orthoses that fabricated for disable persons discussed in the Dollar and Herr review paper, but the effect of advanced powered orthosis on walking in paraplegia patients was not analyzed in their study [39]. Duerinck et al. reported an overview of the influence of the ankle-foot robot-assisted rehabilitation orthoses to the attributes of normal gait in patients with spinal cord injury. They conducted that pneumatic artificial muscles in combination with proportional myoelectric control can restore the attributes of normal gait. In this review, only powered ankle foot orthosis evaluated on walking in SCI patients [40]. Del-Amae et al. reviewed powered gait orthosis that used FES on the muscles as natural actuators to generate gait in persons with spinal cord injury. Their paper explained an overview of hybrid lower limb exoskeletons, related technologies and advances in actuation and control systems, but the efficiency of this type of assistive devices was not evaluated on walking in SCI patients [41].

3. Daily living of spinal cord injury patients

Daily living including independence, orthosis donning and doffing, sitting and standing, walking on slope surfaces and curbs and toileting have been reported in few documents and literatures. Insufficient evidence exists as to the effect of powered and hybrid orthoses on daily living parameters in comparison with mechanical orthosis because these kinds of orthoses have evaluated in laboratory.

About mechanical orthoses, researchers have noted that in comparison to the RGOs, wearing the WO and HGOs has been reported to be easier to don and doff [42, 43]. In comparison between WO and IRGO, the WO has also been demonstrated to provide easier sitting and standing [15]. In comparison between HGO and RGO, it was demonstrated that the HGO has been reported to be easier to don and doff [42]. There are only three documents that analyzed mechanical orthosis on sloped surfaces and have demonstrated that the RGO was slightly more effective than the HGO when SCI subjects were negotiating curbs or slopes [10, 15, 42]. In a comparison between a MLOs and RGOs, the IRGO was significantly better than the WO (p value = 0.03) in 1:12 and 1:26 gradients [15]. It has demonstrated that using the Moorong orthoses in negotiating slopes surfaces was more functional than the WO due to the ability to align the orthotic and anatomic joints [44]. There is no evidence of any significant difference between any types of orthosis with regards to toileting.

Mechanical orthoses have different effects in improvement of parameters, which affect the daily living activities of SCI patients. No study was found, which considered these factors comprehensively in a selection of patients. From an independence view, the light and uncomplicated structure of the MLOs with removable hip joints and without a rigid spinal component made them easier for donning and doffing than RGOs [21, 22, 45]. The lumbar portion of IRGOs compared to MLOs limited the pelvis and lumbar joints. Unlocked joints in the IRGO caused more crutch support. Therefore, wearing IRGOs makes it more difficult than the MLO to provide sitting and standing [15], and additional document is required to demonstrate how assistive devices can help to provide activity of daily living more easily in the SCI patients. Therefore, from independence view, the comparison between MLO and RGO will be beneficial in this field.

4. Energy expenditure of spinal cord injury patients

Excessive energy expenditure and increased applied force on upper limb joints are two most important factors that increase rejection rates of orthoses in paraplegia patients. There are different methods of evaluation of energy expenditure including O_2 cost (ml kg^{-1} m^{-1}), O_2 consumption (ml kg^{-1} min^{-1}), the PCI (beat per m), HR (beat per min), O_2 uptake (l min^{-1}) and the respiratory exchange ratio in SCI patients when using orthoses in all of the documents. However, PCI was introduced as a most sensitive indicator for evaluation of energy expenditure in SCI patients [46]. In other hand, there is little evidence regarding the efficacy of powered gait orthoses (PGOs) and hybrid orthoses when directly compared to mechanical orthoses in reducing energy expenditure in SCI subjects. However, documents have demonstrated that PGOs and hybrid orthoses have less energy expenditure in comparison with mechanical orthoses [5, 47, 48].

SCI patients do not use their mechanical orthoses, with abandonment rates of 61–90% for children with myelomeningocele [49, 50] and 46–54% in adults with spinal cord injury [10, 51–53] due to the high level of energy expenditure needed to ambulate.

One of main reasons for the development of PGOs was to potentially reduce energy consumption when walking with an orthosis. A healthy subject walk with 0.176 mL/kg/m energy expenditure [2] and a SCI subject walk with WBCO 5.41 J/kg/s energy expenditure [54]. The difference between healthy normal subject and walking with a powered orthosis is therefore substantial, but is still improved when compared to that noted when paraplegic subjects walk with mechanical orthoses. There is not enough literature on energy cost of walking with powered orthosis. A further understanding of the energy cost of powered orthosis ambulation is therefore required for patients with SCI.

Kawashima et al., in evaluation of the weight bearing control orthoses on energy consumption stated that the energy consumption of walking has been quoted as being 5.41 J/kg/s [54] for SCI persons, while the mean of this parameter was reported 0.176 mL/kg/m in healthy participants [2]. Arazpour et al. in evaluation of the wearing PGOs compared to the mechanical orthoses such as HKAFO and IRGO reported that wearing PGO provided improved speed of walking and distance walked. The value of the PCI reduced in using the PGO compared to other mechanical orthoses. Active hip and knee joints in providing activated sagittal plane motions were announced as responsible for these results [55]. In a comparison between the WPAL and Primewalk orthoses on energy consumption in four people with paraplegia, Tanabe et al. reported that the PCI exhibited was reduced when using the WPAL [56]. The effort of walking has been shown to be reduced when using a powered motorized ARGO compared to mechanical ARGO in SCI patients [34]. Based on limited studies in evaluation of PGOs on energy consumption in paraplegic patients, a further understanding of this parameter is therefore required for patients with SCI when using PGOs.

About hybrid orthoses, Nene and Patrick [57] in evaluation of using hybrid orthoses (combination of Parawalker and electrical stimulation of the gluteal muscles) in three subjects reported that the rate of the energy cost was 11.78 J/kg/m and 10.95 J/kg/m (a 7.1% reduction) in without functional electrical stimulation (FES) and with FES condition, respectively. Using FES announced a considerable responsibility for reduction in the vertical crutch impulse values (mean 21%) [57]. The lowest energy costs (kcal/kg min) were associated with the RGO and FES, followed by the RGO, HGO, LLB and FES for walking speeds below 28 m/s.

Merati et al. [5] compared the energy cost of locomotion demonstrated by 14 SCI patients (lesion level C7 ± T11) during ambulation with different orthoses (the HGO, Parawalker, RGO and RGO + FES). They observed that during locomotion at maximal speed, HR peak values were 160 ± 16, 155 ± 31 and 154 ± 31 bts/min and VO2 1/kg peak values were 18.0 ± 6.1, 18.5 ± 5.4 and 19.1 ± 7.2 for PW, RGO and RGO + FNS, respectively. During orthosis-assisted locomotion at maximal speed, HR peak values were 150 ± 13, 131 ± 21 and 155 ± 23 bts/min, and VO_2 1/kg peak values were 13.4 ± 3.0, 13.8 ± 3.5 and 17.2 ± 4.8 for PW, RGO and RGO + FNS, respectively. They also reported that maximal ventilations at VO2 peak were 63.8 ± 24.0, 68.9 ± 27.1 and 67.6 ± 23.91 1/min during wheelchair ambulation, and 71.8 ± 7.3, 76.5 ± 21.3 and 72.3 ± 12.2 m/kg/min during orthosis locomotion for PW, RGO and RGO + FNS, respectively [5]. The PEDro score for this study was a 4/10, which equals the highest score assigned in this group.

In mechanical orthoses, connector cable ARGO maintains the posture and reduce PCI and IRGO (2.6 beat/m) has been shown to be more effective than an RGO (3.6 beat/m). Participants in this study reported less fatigue when they used the IRGO [46]. In comparison between RGOs and MLOs, RGOs have less energy expenditure, because MLOs do not have flexion-assist system for the SCI patients and have limited trunk stability, which made patients expend additional effort to maintain upright stance [58]. Also in comparison between MLOs, there is no significant difference in PCI.

RGOs produce less energy expenditure than MLOs and KAFOs [58, 59]. This is because RGOs offer more support for pelvis and trunk and possess a reciprocal system [58]. Energy expenditure and endurance have indirect correlation [60]. Muscle dysfunction, locked position of the ankle and knee joints, flexion of the trunk for providing stability and ambulation with assistive devices such as walker and crutch increase energy consumption in paraplegic subjects in wearing and walking with mechanical orthoses. Ankle and knee joints fixed position can increase energy consumption by up to 33% [60, 61]. Development of the ankle and knee joints of mechanical orthoses via powered or movable structures can be announced as the feasible approach to reduce energy expenditure. The energy consumption of using RGOs reported low rate compared to other mechanical orthoses such as MLOs and HKAFOs, based on the reciprocal section of RGOs announced as the responsible for this result. But the effect of the reciprocal link in providing of the reciprocal motion was demonstrated less [62–64]. Using RGOs for SCI patients rather than MLOs is cumbersome due to their bulky structure and using an MLO has high energy consumption compared to RGOs, but MLOs are more user-friendly for people with SCI [15, 65]. As a result, development of the MLOs with additional structure to provide reciprocal motion announced as the better approach in reduction of the energy expenditure in the SCI subjects. Therefore, the comparison of MLOs and IRGOs on the energy cost, energy expenditure and endurance of the ambulation to provide more effective mechanical orthoses in orthotic rehabilitation of ambulation in the SCI subjects will be important and beneficial.

In comparison between IRGO and RGO on energy consumption in four paraplegic SCI subjects with T3–T12 level of injury, the PCI was reduced when wearing the IRGO (2.6 beat/m), compared to condition that the RGO was used (3.6 beat/m). SCI patients announced less rate of the fatigue while walking with the IRGO [46]. Walking with standard ARGOs demonstrated the reduction of the energy consumption compared to an ARGO without a reciprocal connector cable (5.4 beat/m vs. 5.8 beat/m), although this difference was not statistically significant [66]. The standard ARGO provided best trunk posture in the SCI patients. This positioning is critical and important in the subjects with high level of injury. Evaluation of using WO on five SCI patients demonstrated that energy expenditure was 9.61 (ml/kg/min) [67]. The rate of the O_2 consumption and cost were announced as 13.79 (ml/kg/min) and 1.28 (ml/kg/m), respectively, in walking with standard ARGO in six SCI subjects [68].

5. Temporal spatial parameters

The findings of literature show that there is no high level of document to demonstrate that PGOs are better than mechanical orthoses such as RGOs and HGO in improving temporal spatial gait parameters in SCI subjects. From financial view, the PGOs are so expensive, and also the more orthotic gait training time and effort required providing them functionally. Walking with this type of orthosis does not propose any acceptable improvement in temporal spatial parameters compared to mechanical orthoses. Consequently, more additional attempt on structure of the powered orthoses is required to provide more acceptable powered device for SCI patient wearing and using [69]. There shows to be no significant difference in reported speed of walking subjects in walking with different RGOs in the SCI patients. The following text demonstrates the findings resulted by the literature, which analyzed the effect of common mechanical orthoses on temporal spatial parameters in the SCI patients.

5.1. Stride length

In comparison between the RGO and HGO, there was no significant difference in stride length [67]. In comparison of the standard ARGO with RGO without connector cable, 7% increase in stride length (0.89 vs. 0.83) was reported. Improvement in providing vertical positioning of the trunk by the connector cable announced the main responsible in the standard ARGO [62]. The mean of stride length was reported to be 0.56 m in SCI patients when using the WO [70]. In newly developed orthoses, Genda et al. demonstrated that the hip-ankle-linked orthoses (HALO), increased stride length by 3% compared to the WO (1.03 vs. 1.00 m) [12]. Six percent increased stride length was demonstrated when ankle foot orthosis with dorsiflexion-assist ankle joints were used in the ARGO (0.94 vs. 1 m) compared to the ARGO associated with solid ankle-foot orthosis. In this study, it was claimed that the moveable ankle joint in the ankle-foot orthosis section could improve stride length [71]. When comparing two medial linked orthoses (the Primewalk and Walkabout orthosis). Onogi et al. reported that there was significant difference between them in this parameter and the mean of stride length was increased by 19% [72].

5.2. Cadence

In a comparison between the RGO and the HGO, Whittle et al. reported no significant difference between them in this parameter [70]. However, Winchester et al. announced that although cadence was better in the IRGO than the RGO, there was no significant difference between them [46]. Ijzerman et al. in an evaluation of the effect of a connector cable reported that using an ARGO with a connector cable increased cadence compared to without one, but not significantly (31.3 vs. 30.3 steps/min) [66].

Four studies assessed the cadence in walking with orthoses associated with medial single hip joints in SCI patients. The mean of this parameter was reported as being 70.02 steps/min when using the WO [67] and 50.9 steps/min when walking with any type of medial single hip joints orthosis [73]. Significant difference in cadence between the HALO and PW devices (74.1 vs. 58.9) was reported by Genda et al. [12]. In a recently published study, the mean of cadence demonstrated a significant difference in value (40.8 vs. 48 steps/min, respectively) when using the WO and the PW [72].

5.3. Speed of walking

The mean of speed of walking has been reported to be 0.214 m/s when using the Parawalker orthosis during ambulation by SCI patients [45]. When using the ARGO, the mean of this parameter was 0.16 m/s [68]. The mean of speed of walking was reported to be similar between the HGO and the RGO (0.24 m/s) by Whittle et al. [70]. In comparison between RGOs, the IRGO was shown to produce a higher speed of walking (0.22) compared to a cable-type RGO (0.21), but there was no significant difference between them [46]. When comparing the KAFO and the IRGO, there were significant differences noted between them in this parameter (p = 0.009) [59]. The effect of a connector cable when using the ARGO has no significant effect on improving walking speed when compared to an ARGO without one (0.24 vs. 0.23 m/s) [62].

The effect of PGOs on walking speed, cadence and step length exhibited by SCI subjects is dependent on which joints are actuated in an orthosis (e.g. the hip or knee actuated separately or by being synchronized). Few studies have directly compared these parameters directly between separately or synchronized movement of the hip and knee joint conditions during walking with PGOs.

Kang et al. [74] in evaluation of the powered IRGO (via using pneumatic actuators in the hip joints) compared to a mechanical IRGO after three months orthotic gait training in three SCI subjects reported that evaluated parameters such as walking speed, pelvic tilt, flexion and extension angles of the knee and hip joints, stance and swing phase times improved. Walking speed was increased by 26% and the percentage swing phase during walking was increased by 25% when walking with the PGO.

Powered lower limb orthoses such as the ReWalk powered orthosis (Argo Medical Technologies), the wearable power-assist locomotor (WPAL) and the eLEGS powered orthosis

(Berkeley Bionics) are all examples of commercially developed powered orthoses designed for walking by paraplegic subjects. The Hybrid Assistive Limb (HAL)—6LB which has six electric motors—bilaterally at the hip, knee and ankle joints, the HAL-5 Type-C, which is previous HAL for paraplegia patients, with only four power units are another examples of power lower limb orthosis. Commercially developed HAL has four power units and uses EMG signals of leg to synchronize the motion support with the wearer's movement, but complete paraplegia patients cannot use this version of HAL.

Speed of walking reported difference between mechanical, hybrid and powered gait orthoses. There was statistically significant difference between orthotic walking and walking in healthy subjects. Since walking with powered orthoses (mechanical orthoses that powered with external actuators in the hip or knee joints) needs to keep balance and other assistive devices such as walker or crutch need to activate the powered joints, therefore, the speed of walking is thought to be adversely affected by these conditions. Commercially developed exoskeletons have shown the potential to significantly improve speed of walking.

Since there were some studies about increased step length and cadence in wearing powered gait orthoses during walking, more research in this field is required. The mechanism of the additional external actuator to mechanical orthosis in the powered gait orthoses in improvement of speed of walking needs more research.

5.3.1. Quiet standing

Mechanical orthosis has been analyzed in a few researches in stability by quite standing. Anterior–posterior (AP) and mediolateral (ML) COP displacement in amplitude and velocity of were measured in SCI patients. Baardman evaluated the effect of connector link in ARGO and reported no difference between ARGO with (35.22 mm in AP and 41.72 mm in ML COP displacement) and without (37.94 mm in AP and 34.53 mm in ML direction) cable in quiet standing in stability [62].

In another study, Middleton et al. compared KAFO with and without a single medial linkage on sway amplitude in SCI patients announced that AP sway amplitude when using a single medial linkage with KAFO was half that when wearing a KAFO without it, but in ML direction amplitude there was no significant difference [75]. In a research Abe et al. compared stability with KAFO, RGO and WO and reported significant difference between KAFO with two other orthoses [75].

5.3.2. Performance

Such as other parameters in PGOs there is no document in relation to performance and powered orthoses. About mechanical orthoses, there are three studies in relation to amplitude and velocity of COP displacement. The first study was reported by Baardman et al., which done on cable connector in the ARGO on performance. These researchers reported no effect of connector cable on performance (COP displacement in quite standing) but demonstrated this cable in ARGO can reduce upper limb load [62].

Middleton et al. compared KAFO with and without single medial linkage and announced no significant difference in sway path and amplitude in the A-P direction between them in SCI patients, but use of KAFO with a medial linkage decreased sway amplitude (p = 0.008) and increased M-L direction of sway path (p = 0.021). Therefore, this research proved using a single medial linkage can increase stability and balance in the mediolateral direction [75]. In the third study, Abe et al. demonstrated that sway amplitude was not significantly different between the WO and the RGO but the KAFO had significantly less stability [76].

6. Future research topics in this field

The following topics can be performed in orthotics rehabilitation of the SCI subjects:

- Based on lack of commercial powered and hybrid orthoses, development of these types of assistive orthoses will be beneficial in this field.

- Analysis of the developed commercial powered and hybrid orthoses on energy cost and energy consumption is essential in this field.

- Finding the solution to reduce energy expenditure during ambulation in SCI patients will be beneficial in rehabilitation of orthotic walking in SCI subjects.

- Analysis of energy expenditure between mechanical orthoses, commercial powered and hybrid orthoses is essential before and after the orthotic gait training in SCI subjects.

7. Summary remarks

- Using the powered gait, orthoses reduced the needed effort during ambulation in SCI subjects. Using external actuators in the hip or knee joints with provided active motions in specific joints announced the main reason for these results.

- Powered gait orthoses can be used in the clinical environment for orthotic gait training purposes. Although the positive effect of the orthotic gait training with WBCO on muscle activity in SCI patients was reported, more research is needed to approve any beneficial influence.

- Based on literature, it is concluded that the powered and hybrid orthoses could be announced as effective devices for orthotic rehabilitation of walking in SCI patients to assist to provide their best ambulation.

- Speed of walking reported difference between mechanical, hybrid and powered gait orthoses. There was statistically significant difference between orthotic walking and waling in healthy subjects.

- Since walking with powered orthoses needs to keep balance and other assistive devices such as walker or crutch need to activate the powered joints, therefore, the speed of walking is thought to be adversely affected by these conditions. Commercially developed exoskeletons have shown the potential to significantly improve speed of walking.

Author details

Mokhtar Arazpour*, Monireh Ahmadi Bani, Mohammad Ebrahim Mousavi, Mahmood Bahramizadeh and Mohammad Ali Mardani

*Address all correspondence to: M.Arazpour@yahoo.com

Department of Orthotics and Prosthetics, University of Social Welfare and Rehabilitation Sciences, Tehran, Iran

References

[1] Varma AK, Das A, Wallace IV G, Barry J, Vertegel AA, Ray SK, et al. Spinal cord injury: a review of current therapy, future treatments, and basic science frontiers. Neurochemical Research 2013;38(5):895–905.

[2] Bernardi M, Macaluso A, Sproviero E, Castellano V, Coratella D, Felici F, et al. Cost of walking and locomotor impairment. Journal of Electromyography and Kinesiology 1999;9(2):149–57.

[3] Hirokawa S, Grimm M, Solomonow M, Baratta R, Shoji H, D'ambrosia R. Energy consumption in paraplegic ambulation using the reciprocating gait orthosis and electric stimulation of the thigh muscles. Archives of Physical Medicine and Rehabilitation 1990;71(9):687–94.

[4] Johnson W, Fatone S, Gard S. Walking mechanics of persons who use reciprocating gait orthoses. Journal of Rehabilitation Research and Development 2009;46(3):435.

[5] Merati G, Sarchi P, Ferrarin M, Pedotti A, Veicsteinas A. Paraplegic adaptation to assisted-walking: energy expenditure during wheelchair versus orthosis use. Spinal Cord 2000;38(1):37–44.

[6] Nene A, Hermens H, Zilvold G. Paraplegic locomotion: a review. Spinal Cord 1996;34(9):507–24.

[7] Solomonow M, Baratta R, Shoji H, et al., eds. FES powered locomotion of paraplegics fitted with the LSU reciprocating gait orthoses (RGO). Proceeding of Annual International Conference on IEEE Engineering. Med Biol Soc 1988;10:1672.

[8]   Motlock WM. principles of orthotic management for child and adult paraplegia and clinical experience with the isocentric RGO. Proceeding of 7th world congress of the international society in prosthetic and orthotics 1992; Chicago, p 28.

[9]   Kirtley C, McKay SK, editors. Total design of the "Walkabout": A new paraplegic walking orthosis. In: ISPO Proceedings 7th World Congress, Chicago, Illinois, 1992, June 28-July 3. ISPO p39.

[10]   Middleton J, Fisher W, Davis G, Smith R. A medial linkage orthosis to assist ambulation after spinal cord injury. Prosthetics and Orthotics International 1998;22(3):258–64.

[11]   Saitoh E, Baba M, Sonoda S, Tomita Y, Suzuki M, Hayashi M. A new medial single hip joint for paraplegic walkers. In: Ueda S, Nakamura R, Ishigami S (eds). The Eighth World Congress of International Rehabilitation Medicine Association. Monduzzi Editore: Bologna, Italy 1997, pp 1299–1305.

[12]   Genda E, Oota K, Suzuki Y, Koyama K, Kasahara T. A new walking orthosis for paraplegics: hip and ankle linkage system. Prosthetics and Orthotics International 2004;28(1):69–74.

[13]   Ahmadi Bani M, Arazpour M, Farahmand F, Mousavi ME, Hutchins SW. The efficiency of mechanical orthoses in affecting parameters associated with daily living in spinal cord injury patients: a literature review. Disability and Rehabilitation: Assistive Technology 2014(0):1–8.

[14]   Harvey L, Davis G, Smith M, Engel S. Energy expenditure during gait using the walkabout and isocentric reciprocal gait orthoses in persons with paraplegia. Archives of Physical Medicine and Rehabilitation 1998;79(8):945–9.

[15]   Harvey LA, Smith MB, Davis GM, Engel S. Functional outcomes attained by T9-12 paraplegic patients with the walkabout and the isocentric reciprocal gait orthoses. Archives of Physical Medicine and Rehabilitation 1997;78(7):706–11.

[16]   Bernardi M, Canale I, Castellano V, Di Filippo L, Felici F, Marchetti M. The efficiency of walking of paraplegic patients using a reciprocating gait orthosis. Paraplegia 1995;33(7):409–15.

[17]   Karimi MT. Functional walking ability of paraplegic patients: comparison of functional electrical stimulation versus mechanical orthoses. European Journal of Orthopaedic Surgery & Traumatology 2013;23(6):631–8.

[18]   Shimada Y, Hatakeyama K, Minato T, Matsunaga T, Sato M, Chida S, et al. Hybrid functional electrical stimulation with medial linkage knee-ankle-foot orthoses in complete paraplegics. The Tohoku Journal of Experimental Medicine 2006;209(2):117–23.

[19]   Yang L, Condie D, Granat M, Paul J, Rowley D. Effects of joint motion constraints on the gait of normal subjects and their implications on the further development of hybrid FES orthosis for paraplegic persons. Journal of Biomechanics 1996;29(2):217–26.

[20] Petrofsky J, Smith JB. Physiologic costs of computer-controlled walking in persons with paraplegia using a reciprocating-gait orthosis. Archives of Physical Medicine and Rehabilitation 1991;72(11):890–6.

[21] Arazpour M, Chitsazan A, Hutchins SW, Ghomshe FT, Mousavi ME, Takamjani EE, et al. Design and simulation of a new powered gait orthosis for paraplegic patients. Prosthetics and Orthotics International 2012;36(1):125–30.

[22] Audu ML, To CS, Kobetic R, Triolo RJ. Gait evaluation of a novel hip constraint orthosis with implication for walking in paraplegia. Neural Systems and Rehabilitation Engineering, IEEE Transactions on 2010;18(6):610–8.

[23] Hornby TG, Zemon DH, Campbell D. Robotic-assisted, body-weight-supported treadmill training in individuals following motor incomplete spinal cord injury. Physical Therapy 2005;85(1):52–66.

[24] Colombo G, Joerg M, Schreier R, Dietz V. Treadmill training of paraplegic patients using a robotic orthosis. Journal of Rehabilitation Research and Development 2000;37(6):693–700.

[25] Van Der Salm A, Nene AV, Maxwell DJ, Veltink PH, Hermens HJ, IJzerman MJ. Gait impairments in a group of patients with incomplete spinal cord injury and their relevance regarding therapeutic approaches using functional electrical stimulation. Artificial Organs 2005;29(1):8–14.

[26] Hidler J. What is next for locomotor-based studies? Journal of Rehabilitation Research and Development 2005;42(1):xi.

[27] Harkema SJ, Hurley SL, Patel UK, Requejo PS, Dobkin BH, Edgerton VR. Human lumbosacral spinal cord interprets loading during stepping. Journal of Neurophysiology 1997;77(2):797–811.

[28] Beres-Jones JA, Harkema SJ. The human spinal cord interprets velocity-dependent afferent input during stepping. Brain 2004;127(10):2232–46.

[29] Vukobratovic M, Hristic D, Stojiljkovic Z. Development of active anthropomorphic exoskeletons. Medical and Biological Engineering and Computing 1974;12(1):66–80.

[30] Belforte G, Gastaldi L, Sorli M. Pneumatic active gait orthosis. Mechatronics 2001;11(3): 301–23.

[31] Belforte G, Eula G, Appendino S, Sirolli S. Pneumatic interactive gait rehabilitation orthosis: design and preliminary testing. Proceedings of the Institution of Mechanical Engineers, Part H: Journal of Engineering in Medicine 2011;225(2):158–69.

[32] Kang S, Ryu J, Moon I, Kim K, Mun M. Walker gait analysis of powered gait orthosis for paraplegic. In: Proceedings of world congress on medical physics and biomedical engineering IFMBE, COEX Seoul, Korea, 27 August –1 September 2006, vol. 14, pp. 2889–2891. Springer, 2007.

[33] Ruthenberg B, Wasylewski N, Beard J. An experimental device for investigating the force and power requirements of a powered gait orthosis. Development 1997;34(2):203–13.

[34] Ohta Y, Yano H, Suzuki R, Yoshida M, Kawashima N, Nakazawa K. A two-degree-of-freedom motor-powered gait orthosis for spinal cord injury patients. Proceedings of the Institution of Mechanical Engineers, Part H: Journal of Engineering in Medicine 2007;221(6):629–39.

[35] Arazpour M, Chitsazan A, Hutchins SW, Ghomshe FT, Mousavi ME, Takamjani EE, et al. Evaluation of a novel powered hip orthosis for walking by a spinal cord injury patient: a single case study. Prosthetics and Orthotics International 2012;36(1):105–12.

[36] Arazpour M, Chitsazan A, Hutchins SW, et al. Evaluation of a novel powered hip orthosis for walking by a spinal cord injury patient: a single case study. Prosthet Orthot Int 2012; 36(1): 105–112.

[37] Bogue R. Robotic exoskeletons: a review of recent progress. Industrial Robot: An International Journal 2015;42(1):5–10.

[38] Ferris DP, Sawicki GS, Domingo A. Powered lower limb orthoses for gait rehabilitation. Topics in Spinal Cord Injury Rehabilitation 2005;11(2):34.

[39] Dollar A, Herr H. Lower extremity exoskeletons and active orthoses: challenges and state-of-the-art. Robotics, IEEE Transactions on 2008;24(1):144–58.

[40] Duerinck S, Swinnen E, Beyl P, Hagman F, Jonkers I, Vaes P, et al. The added value of an actuated ankle-foot orthosis to restore normal gait function in patients with spinal cord injury: a systematic review. Journal of Rehabilitation Medicine 2012;44(4):299–309.

[41] Arazpour M, Hutchins SW, Bani MA. The efficacy of powered orthoses on walking in persons with paraplegia. Prosthetics and Orthotics International 2014:0309364613520031.

[42] Whittle M, Cochrane G, Chase A, Copping A, Jefferson R, Staples D, et al. A comparative trial of two walking systems for paralysed people. Paraplegia 1991;29(2):97.

[43] Saitoh E, Suzuki T, Sonoda S, Fujitani J, Tomita Y, Chino N. Clinical experience with a new hip-knee-ankle-foot orthotic system using a medial single hip joint for paraplegic standing and walking 1. American Journal of Physical Medicine & Rehabilitation 1996;75(3):198.

[44] Middleton J, Yeo J, Blanch L, Vare V, Peterson K, Brigden K. Clinical evaluation of a new orthosis, the 'walkabout', for restoration of functional standing and short distance mobility in spinal paralysed individuals. Spinal Cord 1997;35(9):574–9.

[45] Nenel A, Hermensl H, Zilvold G. Paraplegic locomotion: a review. Spinal Cord 1996;34:507–24.

[46] Winchester P, Carollo J, Parekh R, Lutz L, Aston J. A comparison of paraplegic gait performance using two types of reciprocating gait orthoses. Prosthetics and Orthotics International 1993;17(2):101–6.

[47] Nene A, Patrick J. Energy cost of paraplegic locomotion using the ParaWalker—electrical stimulation ``hybrid'' orthosis. Archives of Physical Medicine and Rehabilitation 1990;71(2):116.

[48] Hirokawa S, Grimm M. Energy consumption in paraplegic ambulation using the reciprocating gait orthosis and electric stimulation of the thigh muscles. Archives of Physical Medicine and Rehabilitation 1990;71(9):687.

[49] Katz-Leurer M, Weber C, Smerling-Kerem J, Rottem H, Meyer S. Prescribing the reciprocal gait orthosis for myelomeningocele children: a different approach and clinical outcome. Pediatric Rehabilitation 2004;7(2):105–9.

[50] Sykes L, Edwards J, Powell ES, Ross ERS. The reciprocating gait orthosis: long-term usage patterns. Archives of Physical Medicine and Rehabilitation 1995;76(8):779–83.

[51] Franceschini M, Baratta S, Zampolini M, Loria D, Lotta S. Reciprocating gait orthoses: a multicenter study of their use by spinal cord injured patients. Archives of Physical Medicine and Rehabilitation 1997;78(6):582–6.

[52] Scivoletto G, Petrelli A, Di Lucente L, Giannantoni A, Fuoco U, D'Ambrosio F, et al. One year follow up of spinal cord injury patients using a reciprocating gait orthosis: preliminary report. Spinal Cord 2000;38(9):555–8.

[53] Jaspers P, Peeraer L, Van Petegem W, Van der Perre G. The use of an advanced reciprocating gait orthosis by paraplegic individuals: a follow-up study. Spinal Cord 1997;35(9):585–9.

[54] Kawashima N, Sone Y, Nakazawa K, Akai M, Yano H. Energy expenditure during walking with weight-bearing control (WBC) orthosis in thoracic level of paraplegic patients. Spinal Cord 2003;41(9):506–10.

[55] Arazpour M, Bani M, Hutchins S, Jones R. The physiological cost index of walking with mechanical and powered gait orthosis in patients with spinal cord injury. Spinal Cord 2013;51(5):356–9.

[56] Tanabe S, Saitoh E, Hirano S, Katoh M, Takemitsu T, Uno A, et al. Design of the Wearable Power-Assist Locomotor (WPAL) for paraplegic gait reconstruction. Disability and Rehabilitation: Assistive Technology 2013;8(1):84–91.

[57] Nene A, Patrick J. Energy cost of paraplegic locomotion with the ORLAU ParaWalker. Spinal Cord 1989;27(1):5–18.

[58] Harvey LA, Davis GM, Smith MB, Engel S. Energy expenditure during gait using the walkabout and isocentric reciprocal gait orthoses in persons with paraplegia. Archives of Physical Medicine and Rehabilitation 1998;79(8):945–9.

[59]   Leung AK, Wong AF, Wong EC, Hutchins SW. The physiological cost index of walking with an isocentric reciprocating gait orthosis among patients with T12–L1 spinal cord injury. Prosthetics and Orthotics International 2009;33(1):61–8.

[60]   Waters RL, Mulroy S. The energy expenditure of normal and pathologic gait. Gait & Posture 1999;9(3):207–31.

[61]   Kerrigan DC, Viramontes BE, Corcoran PJ, LaRaia PJ. Measured versus predicted vertical displacement of the sacrum during gait as a tool to measure biomechanical gait performance. American Journal of Physical Medicine & Rehabilitation 1995;74(1):3–8.

[62]   Baardman G, Ijzerman M, Hermen H, Veltink P, Boom H, Zilvold G. The influence of the reciprocal hip joint link in the Advanced Reciprocating Gait Orthosis on standing performance in paraplegia. Prosthetics and Orthotics International 1997;21(3):210–21.

[63]   Dall P, Müller B, Stallard I, Edwards J, Granat M. The functional use of the reciprocal hip mechanism during gait for paraplegic patients walking in the Louisiana State University reciprocating gait orthosis. Prosthetics and Orthotics International 1999;23(2):152–62.

[64]   Johnson WB, Fatone S, Gard SA. Walking mechanics of persons who use reciprocating gait orthoses. Journal of Rehabilitation Research and & Development 2009;46(3): 435–46.

[65]   Harvey LA, Newton-John T, Davis GM, Smith MB, Engel S. A comparison of the attitude of paraplegic individuals to the walkabout orthosis and the isocentric reciprocal gait orthosis. Spinal Cord 1997;35(9):580–4.

[66]   Ijzerman M, Baardman G, Hermens H, Veltink P, Boom H, Zilvold G. The influence of the reciprocal cable linkage in the advanced reciprocating gait orthosis on paraplegic gait performance. Prosthetics and Orthotics International 1997;21(1):52–61.

[67]   Saitoh E, Suzuki T, Sonoda S, Fujitani J, Tomita Y, Chino N. Clinical experience with a new hip-knee-ankle-foot orthotic system using a medial single hip joint for paraplegic standing and walking 1. American Journal of Physical Medicine & Rehabilitation 1996;75(3):198–203.

[68]   Massucci M, Brunetti G, Piperno R, Betti L, Franceschini M. Walking with the advanced reciprocating gait orthosis (ARGO) in thoracic paraplegic patients: energy expenditure and cardiorespiratory performance. Spinal Cord 1998;36(4):223–7.

[69]   Arazpour M, Bani MA, Hutchins SW. Reciprocal gait orthoses and powered gait orthoses for walking by spinal cord injury patients. Prosthetics and Orthotics International 2013;37(1):14–21.

[70]   Whittle M, Cochrane G, Chase A, Copping A, Jefferson R, Staples D, et al. A comparative trial of two walking systems for paralysed people. Spinal Cord 1991;29(2):97–102.

[71]   Bani MA, Arazpour M, Ghomshe FT, Mousavi ME, Hutchins SW. Gait evaluation of the advanced reciprocating gait orthosis with solid versus dorsi flexion assist ankle foot

orthoses in paraplegic patients. Prosthetics and Orthotics International 2013;37(2):161–7.

[72] Onogi K, Kondo I, Saitoh E, Kato M, Oyobe T. Comparison of the effects of sliding-type and hinge-type joints of knee-ankle-foot orthoses on temporal gait parameters in patients with paraplegia. Japanese Journal of Comprehensive Rehabilitation Science 2010;1:1–6.

[73] Suzuki T, Sonoda S, Saitoh E, Onogi K, Fujino H, Teranishi T, et al. Prediction of gait outcome with the knee–ankle–foot orthosis with medial hip joint in patients with spinal cord injuries: a study using recursive partitioning analysis. Spinal Cord 2007;45(1):57–63.

[74] Middleton JW, Sinclair PJ, Smith RM, Davis GM. Postural control during stance in paraplegia: effects of medially linked versus unlinked knee-ankle-foot orthoses. Archives of Physical Medicine and Rehabilitation 1999;80(12):1558–65.

[75] Abe K. Comparison of static balance, walking velocity, and energy consumption with knee-ankle-foot orthosis, walkabout orthosis, and reciprocating gait orthosis in thoracic-level paraplegic patients. JPO: Journal of Prosthetics and Orthotics 2006;18(3):87–91.

8

Experimental Spinal Cord Injury Models in Rodents: Anatomical Correlations and Assessment of Motor Recovery

Christina F. Vogelaar and Veronica Estrada

Abstract

Human traumatic spinal cord injury (SCI) causes disruption of descending motor and ascending sensory tracts, which leads to severe disturbances in motor functions. To date, no standard therapy for the regeneration of severed spinal cord axons in humans exists. Experimental SCI in rodents is essential for the development of new treatment strategies and for understanding the underlying mechanisms leading to motor recovery. Here, we provide an overview of the main rodent models and techniques available for the investigation of neuronal regeneration and motor recovery after experimental SCI.

Keywords: spinal cord injury, regeneration, plasticity, rodent, motor recovery

1. Introduction

The challenge of spinal cord injury (SCI) research is to find the right model for testing new treatment strategies. Although rodents differ from humans in many aspects, the research on primates is prohibited in many countries, and there are very strict regulations on experimenting with nonhuman primates [1]. Therefore, rodent models are the first choice for testing the effectiveness and mechanisms of new potential treatments for SCI. Rodents, especially mice, provide the additional advantage of transgenic technologies (knock out and knock in) that can be helpful in SCI research. In this chapter, an extensive description is provided on the currently available rodent SCI models, methods of treatment application, histological analysis of regenerating axons, and functional analysis of motor recovery.

2. Anatomy of the longitudinal axon tracts in rodents and humans

In order to understand the impact of SCI, it is important to have some basic knowledge about the long axon tracts that are interrupted by the lesion. Descending tracts control various motor functions. Sensory information from ascending tracts is also essential for posture, balance, and coordination of movements. Here, the main projections from the brain to the spinal cord and vice versa are summarized.

2.1. Descending motor tracts

The descending tracts in the spinal cord (**Figure 1**, left-hand side) run from the brain and brainstem to the spinal cord and are all involved in motor control [2].

2.1.1. Corticospinal tract (CST)

The corticospinal tract (CST) is variable between species. The motor cortex in rodents, generally referred to as the sensorimotor cortex (a rostrocaudal gradient of motor and sensory areas), is not as well defined as it is in humans, who have separate areas for sensory and motor cortex. The CST is responsible for the control of fine movements of distal musculature (e.g., fingers). Pyramidal neurons in layer V of the motor area give rise to the corticospinal axons that run via the internal capsule to the brainstem pyramids where they cross. It then depends on the species which path the majority of CST axons follow. In primates, almost all crossed fibers run in the lateral CST, located in the dorsolateral part of the lateral column. In rodents, most fibers are located in the dorsal CST (dCST), running in the ventral part of the dorsal columns. In some species, a ventral CST (vCST) is also observed. The CST axons terminate mainly in lamina 3–6 of the grey matter. In humans, up to 20% of CST axons terminate directly on motoneurons in lamina 9. CST terminals are glutamatergic.

2.1.2. Rubrospinal tract (RST)

The rubrospinal tract (RST) plays a role in general locomotion and in some species controls more skilled motor tasks together with the CST. It arises from the caudal magnocellular part of the red nucleus and crosses in the ventral tegmental decussation. The RST descends in the dorsal part of the spinal cord lateral column. The axons terminate in laminae 5 and 6 (sometimes 7) in the cervical and lumbosacral enlargements corresponding to the limbs. In rats, direct termination on lamina 9 motoneurons has been reported. The RST is prominent in rodents, whereas in animals with a large lateral CST (e.g., primates and humans), the RST is smaller. RST axons use glutamate as neurotransmitter.

2.1.3. Reticulospinal tracts (ReST)

The reticular formation in the brainstem plays a role in the preparation of movements and postural control. Reticulospinal tracts run medially and laterally in the ventral part of the spinal cord white matter. Whereas the medial reticulospinal tract (ReST) remains uncrossed, part of the lateral ReST fibers cross to the contralateral side. The ReST does not form a clear bundle but intermingles with fibers from other tracts, for example, the vestibulospinal and spinotha-lamic tracts. The axons terminate in laminae 5–9 and can be either glutamatergic or GABAergic [3].

2.1.4. Vestibulospinal tracts (VeST)

The medial and lateral vestibulospinal tracts (VeSTs) are responsible for the initiation of limb and trunk extensor activity, which is important for posture. The lateral VeST arises from the lateral vestibular nucleus and does not cross, whereas the medial VeST originates from both the medial and the spinal vestibular nuclei and partially crosses to the contralateral side. Both run in the ventral white matter and terminate in laminae 7–8, providing glutamatergic input [3].

2.1.5. Raphespinal and coeruleospinal tracts

The Raphe nuclei give rise to the raphespinal projections, which together with the coeruleo-spinal projections (from the locus coeruleus) modulate (among others) motor functions. The raphespinal projections include a non-serotonergic component that runs in the dorsolateral funiculus and is involved in gating pain, as well as a serotonergic component that runs in the ventrolateral white matter, terminating in the intermediate grey and on motoneurons in the ventral horn. The noradrenergic coeruleospinal fibers run without crossing in the ventral funiculus and project throughout the grey matter.

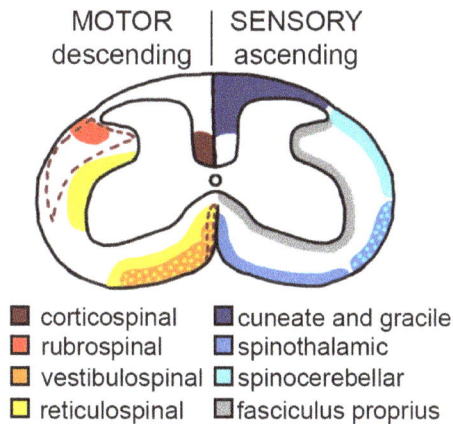

Figure 1. Spinal cord anatomy: schematic representation of the main ascending sensory tracts (right) and descending motor tracts (left) in a transverse section of the rodent spinal cord. Dotted areas represent locations where tracts are intermingled. Dashed lines indicate the location of the corticospinal tract in humans.

2.2. Ascending sensory tracts

The ascending tracts in the spinal cord (**Figure 1**, right-hand side) convey sensory information from the periphery to central nervous system (CNS) areas involved in walking, posture, and information processing about noxious stimuli [4].

2.2.1. Gracile and cuneate tracts

These two large ascending pathways contain axons from the dorsal root ganglia (DRGs) and provide sensory information from the limbs and trunk. In rodents, an additional dorsal column nucleus contains afferent axons from the tail. The tracts synapse in the gracile and cuneate nuclei located in the medulla oblongata. The second-order axons then cross the midline and run through the medial lemniscus to the thalamus. A subpopulation of DRG neurons synapses locally on dorsal horn neurons, whose axons also project to the gracile and cuneate nuclei. This is called the post-synaptic dorsal column pathway, whereas those DRG axons that do not synapse locally constitute the direct dorsal column pathway.

2.2.2. Spinothalamic, spinoreticular, and spinovestibular tracts

Several sensory tracts run in the ventrolateral funiculus of the spinal cord. These include the spinothalamic tract that conveys nociceptive, thermal, crude touch, and pressure information from the DRGs to the thalamus. The spinoreticular tract provides pain information to brainstem nuclei of the reticular formation. The spinovestibular tract is important for bringing proprioceptive signals to the vestibular nuclei. Several other tracts are present in the ventrolateral funiculus, such as the spinomesencephalic, spinoparabrachial, spinohypothalamic, and spinocervical tracts, each providing information to specific brain regions, that is, mesencephalon, parabrachial nuclei, hypothalamus, and lateral cervical nucleus in the upper cervical cord, respectively.

2.2.3. Spinocerebellar tracts

Projection axons from the spinal cord to the cerebellum are located in the dorsolateral and ventrolateral funiculi (**Figure 1** right-hand side). They carry proprioceptive information from the muscles and tendons to the cerebellum, so that adjustments of posture and coordination of movements can take place.

2.3. The propriospinal system

The spinal cord's "own" projection system refers to neurons that are located in the spinal cord, whose axons interconnect various spinal cord levels [5]. This so-called propriospinal system constitutes a large part of the white matter. It comprises interneurons that are connected to either other interneurons or directly to motoneurons. With respect to locomotor control, short-axon propriospinal neurons are also called premotoneurons, because they modulate corticospinal and sensory input to motoneuron pools controlling fore- and hindlimb activity. The long-axon propriospinal neurons form connections between the cervical and lumbosacral enlargements and are responsible for coordination of fore- and hindlimbs. These axons run in the fasciculus proprius (**Figure 1**, right-hand side).

The propriospinal neurons also modulate input to the lumbar central pattern generator (CPG), a local system involved in reflexive stepping in total absence of supraspinal input [5]. Serotonin from brainstem neurons has been shown to play a major role in CPG activation [6, 7].

3. Rodent spinal cord injury models

The choice of SCI models is important in view of comparability with human SCI, but practical issues should also be considered. Although human lesions are usually compressions (but some may be sharp wounds as well or a mixture of both), from the experimental point of view it might be important to have a more "clean" and reproducible cut. Treatment strategies that fail to cause regeneration through a spinal cord transection lesion will probably have equally small effects after contusion lesions. On the contrary, treatments that induce regeneration in a transection model should then be tested and optimized in a contusion model. Partial injury models are useful for the investigation of the locomotor recovery over time, since not only regeneration but also sprouting from spared axon tracts can occur (see Section 5). Models of complete transection are used to study regeneration without the possibility of plasticity processes bypassing the lesion. While the complete transection of the spinal cord is a very reproducible injury, disadvantages of this lesion model are the poor degree of regenerative

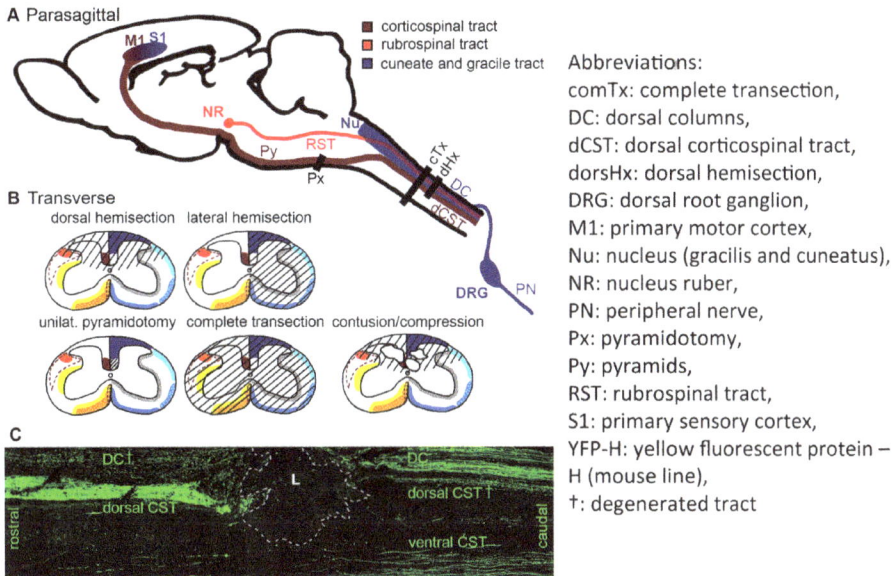

Figure 2 Spinal cord lesions in rodent models of SCI: (A) schematic representation of a parasagittal section through the brain and spinal cord (modified from Paxinos & Watson, The Rat Brain in Stereotaxic Coordinates, 6th Edition). Tracts with clear localizations are indicated. It should be noted that these do not run in the same spinal cord section, with the RST (red) running more laterally than the CST (brown) and the cuneate and gracile tracts (blue). The dorsal hemisection, complete transection, and the pyramidotomy lesions are represented as black bars. (B) Schematic drawings of transverse sections through the spinal cord with bilateral motor tracts depicted left and bilateral sensory tracts depicted right (for exact description of the tracts see **Figure 1**). Dashed areas represent the extent of tissue damage produced by the different injury paradigms. Note that motor and sensory tracts run in both spinal cord hemispheres but are depicted separately for better understanding. (C) Histological parasagittal section through the spinal cord of YFP-H mice (The Jackson Laboratory) 7 days after a dorsal hemisection (compilation of 2 sagittal sections). Descending CST axons are intact rostrally and have degenerated caudally from the lesion site (dashed white line). Ventral CST fibers are not lesioned (plane of section causes apparent lack rostrally). Ascending dorsal column axons are intact caudally and have degenerated rostrally.

growth of the severed axons and the general inadequacy for most motor tests. In this section, the technical principles of each model in rats and mice are described.

3.1. Dorsal hemisection (Hx)

Spinal cord transection lesions are generally applied using scissors, scalpel blades, or fine retractable wire knives. The advantage of wire knives (McHugh Millieux) is that a SCI can be performed with high precision, because they can be attached to a stereotactic frame. The dorsal Hx (Figure 2A–C) is the most used SCI paradigm for the investigation of the regeneration of CST and, depending on the extent of lateral lesion, it also includes the RST. It is mostly performed at thoracic level 8 (T8) and involves the laminectomy at T8-9, opening of the dura mater and subsequent lesioning of the spinal cord [8, 9]. For mice, microdissection spring scissors (Fine Science Tools) are used to hemisect the spinal cord. Since this procedure is inherently variable, the experimenter needs to test various depths to determine the desired extension of the lesion. A more controlled technique for dorsal Hx in mice was described by Hill et al. (2009) who used a so-called Vibraknife (LISA-Vibraknife; Louisville, KY) [10, 11]. Dorsal hemisection lesions are usually applied at thoracic spinal cord levels and result in the formation of a dense inhibitory scar [12, 13]. Depending on the severity of the lesion, the animals spontaneously recover a certain degree of walking that can be further ameliorated by regeneration promoting treatments.

3.2. Lateral Hx

For lateral Hx, the lateral half of the spinal cord is transected in mostly the same technical procedure as the dorsal Hx, with the difference that the tracts on one side are left intact (Figure 2B). These lesions provide the advantage of an internal control situation [14], which is also reflected in the behavioral testing, where paw preferences are often scored (see Section 7.5.). Lateral Hx experiments are usually performed at cervical levels, allowing the analysis of both fore- and hindlimb recovery. Mostly, a lesion at cervical level C5 is produced, but some groups have specialized on the analysis of breathing musculature after a lesion at C2 [15].

3.3. Complete transection (Tx)

For a complete transection (Figure 2B), small scissors are generally used to transect the spinal cord after having cut the meninges. Alternatively, the dura mater is opened just enough to allow the insertion of a spinal cord hook (Fine Science Tools) between dura and spinal cord. The hook is then used to lift the cord in order to completely cut the spinal cord. The dura mater can be closed with fine sutures (10-O) after the procedure. The complete Tx model is useful to investigate the effect of treatments on the axonal regeneration, and on (limited) recovery of locomotor function. After a complete SCI in rats, there is usually the development of fluid-filled cavities, whereas in mice this is generally not the case [16].

3.4. Contusion and compression injury

Contusion injuries are the most widely used lesion type in SCI research, since the majority of human SCI involves a contusion or compression pathology. Several commercially available systems can be used to inflict standardized graded contusion injuries. These include the NYU MASCIS impactor (New York University Multicenter Animal SCI Study) [17], the OSU impactor (Ohio State University electromagnetic SCI device) [18, 19], the IH impactor (Infinite Horizon) [20], and the spinal cord compression device (Kopf Instruments). In general, a controlled pressure is exerted on the spinal cord after laminectomy by either dropping or placing a weight onto the cord, controlling the force and/or velocity [21]. Depending on the species (in rats more than in mice), contusion injury leads to cyst formation (Figure 2B), a feature also displayed by human SCI patients [19, 21]. Thoracic contusions are usually performed to induce dorsal bilateral lesions, whereas contusions at the cervical level are performed unilaterally [20].

Compression/decompression models are frequently used to investigate the occlusion of the central canal, another common symptom of SCI in human patients. To perform an experimental compression, injury clips, balloons, or forceps are widely used [21]. Vascular clips and calibrated forceps can be used to create graded and reproducible injuries. The clip compression model and the contusion injury model show some resemblances as they both inflict the injury via pressure to the outer surface of the spinal cord. These models can be fine-tuned so that injuries of varying degrees can be created. They lead to the formation of fluid-filled cysts which are surrounded by spared tissue. The remaining tissue continuity and axon sparing makes them also a suitable model for locomotor functional tests. For the same reason, however, SCI contusion and compression models are not as well suited as transection models to investigate the neuronal and axonal regeneration.

3.5. Pyramidotomy

An exclusive CST-only lesion can be achieved by pyramidotomy, a transection at the height of the pyramids [22] (Figure 2A–B). The injury of the CST by pyramidotomy does not greatly affect locomotion in rodents. Rats and mice use the CST primarily for fine finger movements, which is greatly relevant for human patients. For the study of motor recovery, specific forepaw tests are used (see Section 7.5.). Since this lesion is usually performed unilaterally, the intact side serves as an internal control and is also used for studying plasticity-related regeneration mechanisms [23].

3.6. New SCI models

Scientists are continuously looking for models that resemble the human injuries more closely. For example, two recent studies focused on lumbosacral SCI, a type of injury affecting an estimated one-third of patients [24, 25]. A model combining SCI and traumatic brain injury was recently introduced, because a proportion of SCI patients additionally suffer from head injuries, for example, due to traffic or diving accidents [26]. Finally, a recent publication on a closed-body SCI by applying a high-pressure air blast in mice provides a model resembling human traumatic SCI [27].

4. The application of treatments

After the choice of the appropriate lesion model for therapy development, the next decision in experimental SCI is the technique to use to apply a treatment. The application method determines the timing, frequency, and duration of the treatment. This section provides technical details of current methods for applying treatments in the various SCI models.

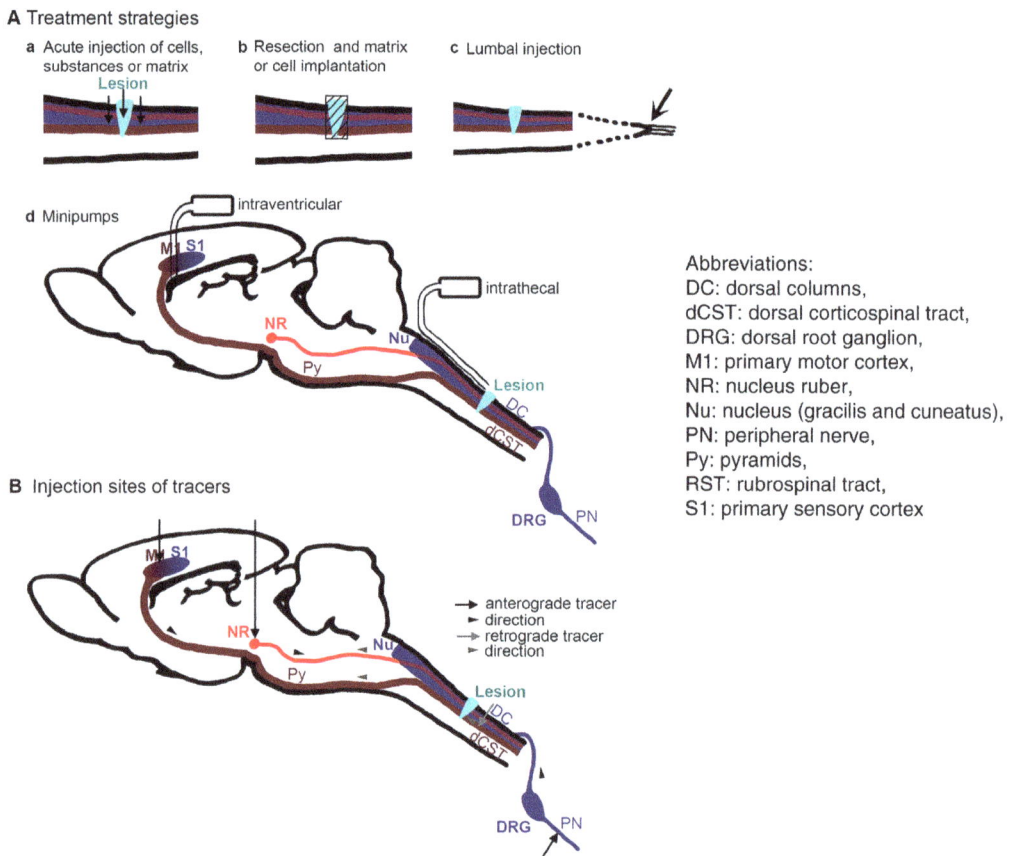

Figure 3 Strategies for the application of treatments and tracers exemplified in a schematic drawing of a dorsal Hx lesion: (A) treatments can be applied by (a) injection into the lesion site and/or adjacent tissue, (b) resection of the chronic lesion scar and subsequent matrix or cell implantation, (c) intrathecal lumbar injection, and (d) infusion over prolonged periods with minipumps and catheters either intraventricularly, intrathecally, or epidurally. The epidural catheter can be guided not only from rostral direction through the cisterna magna but also from the caudal side by performing an additional laminectomy [9, 28]. (B) Anterograde tracers are injected into the motor cortex and nucleus ruber in order to label CST and RST, respectively, and in the peripheral nerve to label the dorsal column axons. Injection of a retrograde tracer caudally to the lesion site is applied in order to visualize the cell bodies corresponding to regenerated axons or local interneuron circuits.

4.1. Injection into the spinal cord parenchyma

The simplest method for acutely applying a therapy is the (single) injection of a substance at the time of surgery. In some models, such as the dorsal Hx, the lesion site is open, so the treatment might potentially diffuse too quickly out of the area. Therefore, treatments are often injected in the intact tissue immediately adjacent to the lesion (Figure 3Aa). The injection volume should not be too high (<1 µl), and the injection should be performed slowly so that additional damage to the tissue is avoided. Controlled injection is achieved either by using a pump (e.g., the Pump 11 Elite Nanomite, Harvard Sachs Elektronik) or by introducing a delay of several minutes between injection and retraction of the needle. The injection method is most suitable for single acute treatments, because any additional doses will require additional surgery.

4.2. Lumbar injection into the CSF

A therapeutic can be applied to the CSF by lumbar intrathecal injection (Figure 3Ac), described in detail for mice by Lu et al, 2013. Shortly, the animal is subjected to a brief inhalation narcosis and kept in half-sleep by keeping its head in a dark environment. The L5 vertebra can be localized between the iliac crests of the hip bones. A 30-gauge needle is used to puncture the skin and enter the spine between the L5 and L6 spinous process. When the dura mater is punctured, a reflective flick of the tail is induced and up to 5 µl liquid can be applied [29]. This method is useful for renewing treatments multiple times after the initial injection.

4.3. Intrathecal application via minipumps

For continuous long-term application of liquid therapeutics, the use of minipumps is a standard delivery method (Figure 3Ad). Pumps can be implanted subcutaneously and attached to a catheter for intrathecal delivery. Minipumps either release the liquid via osmosis (Alzet®) or they use a programmable microprocessor (iPrecio®). They are commercially available in different sizes and with varying pumping rates and time periods. The subcutaneously placed minipumps can be removed after the required delivery period. The minipumps are connected to a catheter which can be inserted in the brain for intraventricular infusion [30], or the catheter can be guided through the epidural space underneath the vertebrae toward the lesion site [19, 28]. It is important to consider that the catheter by itself can produce a compression of the spinal cord. This is especially problematic in mice, because of their size, although special mouse catheters are available commercially (Alzet®).

4.4. Cellular transplantation strategies

Cell therapy is generally the focus in neurodegenerative diseases such as Alzheimer's or Parkinson's disease where the common goal is to replace degenerated neurons. In contrast, SCI is characterized by damage of the neuronal processes, whereas the corresponding cell bodies are located in various areas of the brain, brainstem, and DRGs, thus complicating cell replacement. Moreover, the projection neurons are thought to undergo atrophy in contrast to dying [31]. Therefore, cellular therapeutic approaches for experimental SCI concentrate on the spinal cord, where local cells are affected by the primary and secondary injury events. The therapies on the one hand aim to replace glial cells or local neurons. Peripheral nerve grafts or Schwann cell cables have been used to bridge the lesion [32, 33]. Transplanted oligodendrocyte precursor cells or Schwann cells have been shown to remyelinate axons, whereas olfactory ensheathing or mucosal cells may provide axon guidance and trophic support [34–36]. Cell therapies using embryonic stem cells, neural stem/progenitor cells, or induced pluripotent stem (iPS) cells mostly aim to provide local pools of neurons that might serve as relay stations, analogue to propriospinal neurons [37–40]. Stem cells might also differentiate into glial cells that can remyelinate axons. On the other hand, stem cells can bridge the lesion gap and promote regeneration by the secretion of trophic factors, the support of angiogenic events, or the inhibition of glutamate toxicity. These effects have been reported for mesenchymal stem cells, bone marrow mesenchymal stromal cells, or unrestricted somatic stem cells from umbilical cord blood [41–43].

The transplantation of (stem) cells is usually performed by injection of cell suspensions into the spinal cord parenchyma (Figure 3Aa). This can be performed acutely by injecting cells into the intact tissue adjacent to the lesion. Alternatively, the lesion is allowed to form over a certain time period (usually 7 days, also called subacute), and a new surgery is performed to inject the cells directly into the lesion site. Factors to consider are cell survival, migration, differentiation into neural/glial cell types, axon outgrowth, and synaptic contacts in the case of neuronal transplants and secretion of regeneration-supportive factors in the case of nonneural transplants.

4.5. Implantation of matrices

Although many studies have proven the beneficial effects of autologous or heterologous cellular grafts in acute and chronic SCI models in animals [44, 45], the use of cell transplantation in human patients often remains a controversial issue [46, 47]. The search for artificial biomaterials for the implantation into the injured spinal cord has been prompted due to the limited access to autologous donor material and immunological problems associated with allograft rejection.

Cavities or cysts that often form after SCI are a major obstacle impeding axonal regeneration. Therefore, the reconnection across the trauma cavity by means of scaffolds or matrices is a major focus in SCI research. In order to provide a favorable growth substrate for regenerating axons, a bridging material should provide and combine several structural, physicochemical, and molecular properties [48]. Materials should ideally be easily modifiable, serve as a scaffold for matrix molecules and/or cellular transplants, and further be immunologically inert and absorbable [49]. Positive results with acellular matrices have been obtained in numerous studies [45, 49–55]. Important advances have recently been reported in the development of biosynthetic conduits for spinal cord repair. Biosynthetic conduits equipped with ECM molecules and different cell lines, and supplemented with neurotrophic growth factors, have been shown to yield encouraging results in the treatment of experimental SCI [51].

In chronic SCI, cavity formation has occurred and a lesion scar has formed, which presents a stable physical and molecular barrier to axonal regeneration. Cavities and sites of scar resection can be treated with bridging or scaffolding materials. Interesting effects were achieved with a polyethylene glycol (PEG) treatment in a chronic SCI paradigm [56]. PEG was used to fill the cavity that was created by resection of the 5-week-old lesion scar in spinal cord-injured rats (Figure 3Ab). After 8 months, long-distance axonal regeneration through and beyond the graft was observed. The PEG matrix was repopulated by blood vessels, astrocytes, and Schwann cells, the latter remyelinating bundles of regenerating axons. These histological parameters were accompanied by long-lasting functional motor improvement. This study suggests that the chronically lesioned tracts are still able to regenerate when provided with the right extracellular environment [56].

4.6. Implantation of a mechanical microconnector system

Complete transections result in a gap between the two spinal cord stumps. Recently, a novel and unique connector device was described [57]. The purpose of this mechanical microconnector system is to reconnect severed spinal cord tissue stumps in the submillimeter range. The microconnector consists of two elliptical discs lined with numerous honeycombed holes. After implantation into the injured rat spinal cord, the device is connected to a vacuum pump, and the tissue stumps are brought into close apposition via the application of negative pressure. The connector discs have a rough surface, allowing the adherence of the spinal cord tissue. Additional features of the mechanical microconnector system are an internal canal system and an inlet tube, which can be connected either to a syringe or to an osmotic minipump to achieve application of therapeutics into the lesion area. Even the implantation of the device alone was sufficient for axon regeneration and led to a significant improvement of locomotor function following complete transection of the thoracic spinal cord [57].

4.7. Electrical stimulation and neuroprothesis

Electric field stimulation has been shown to promote enhanced and/or oriented neurite outgrowth, thereby offering potential additional treatment strategies after PNS but also CNS injury [58–60]. For SCI treatment, epidural stimulation has been used to create electric fields to restore motor functions [61, 62]. Electrical current is applied at varying frequencies and intensities to the areas of the lumbosacral spinal cord, activating the CPG. The CPG can initiate stepping function even without any input from the brain. The lab of Grégoire Courtine developed a neuroprosthetic that achieves a high-fidelity control of leg kinematics. A closed-loop system, using muscle activity and other kinematic parameters in real-time to feed back into the system, allowed neuromodulation during walking [63]. Another study used neuro-prosthetic intervention in the form of a Neurochip 2 recurrent brain-computer interface in a cervical hemisection model. The neurochip delivered electrical stimulation and measured in parallel the electromyographic (EMG) activity of the muscles, thus adjusting the stimulation according to the muscle activity. Animals that received this so-called targeted, activity-dependent stimulation displayed increased skilled forepaw reaching as compared to animals receiving non-targeted stimulations or physical training [64].

Although it has no direct effect on the regeneration of axons after SCI, epidural stimulation is a very promising approach already used for the rehabilitation of SCI patients with promising results [65].

4.8. Exercise and training

The first studies suggesting that exercise might stimulate motor recovery were performed using environment enrichment [66, 67]. During the last decades, several investigators developed new experimental settings to perform motor training of animals. For example, forced walking on treadmills, training either bipedal or quadrupedal stepping, has been shown to improve locomotor recovery after SCI [68–70]. The combination of treadmill training with epidural stimulation and the administration of serotonergic and dopaminergic agonists seemed to be especially effective in restoring motor activity. Extensive plasticity of corticospinal, brainstem, and intraspinal connectivity was shown to underlie the observed functional recovery [61].

Recently, Starkey et al. (2015) developed a new type of cage with enriched environment over three floors with different types of training possibilities (e.g., grasping tasks, ladder walking, and climbing). This so-called "natural habitat cage" was combined with a new three-dimensional animal tracking system to allow high-impact, self-motivated training. Interestingly, differences were observed between the animals' overall activity and preference for certain tasks. Healthy as well as SCI animals trained in these cages performed better in experimental tests for fine motor control of fore- and hindlimb [71]. For forelimb training, a robotic rehabilitation system was recently developed, in which the animal has to pull a bar to receive food. This setup could also be used to measure forelimb strength [72].

4.9. Other types of treatments

Systemic treatments (intravenous, intraperitoneal, subcutaneous) are not discussed above, although they are clinically relevant. For treatments outside the spinal column, it should in general be known whether the applied therapeutic can cross the blood-brain barrier. A much higher concentration must be applied peripherally to achieve an effective concentration centrally. Since human SCI almost invariably involves surgery, the possibility of local treatment is given.

4.10. Combination treatments

It has become more and more apparent that combination therapies will be necessary to successfully treat SCI. The above described matrices, cell transplantations, electrical stimulation, and training paradigms all offer possibilities of combination with trophic factors, pharmacological treatments, agonists or antagonists of neurotransmitters, anti-inhibitory treatments, and so forth. It seems likely that holistic treatments combining several regeneration mechanisms will be clinically more successful to target the multitude of SCI systems.

5. Possible treatment effects on neurons

5.1. Regeneration versus sprouting

For researchers, the "holy grail" is the regeneration of the injured fibers through the lesion scar and the subsequent reinnervation of their targets. After an initial retraction phase, the axons of the above-described tracts usually start regrowing toward the lesion site. Treatments can increase the regenerative growth of various tracts through and beyond the lesion site [73]. Although this process could be called "sprouting," it is important to distinguish between regenerative sprouting of the severed tract with the goal of regrowth toward the original connections and plastic sprouting, with the goal to find alternatives routes (**Figure 4**). Functional recovery of locomotion can also be achieved through plasticity of intact fibers that may form contralateral sprouts or make new synapses with local propriospinal neurons (**Figure 4**). In the last decade, the propriospinal system became a major focus for SCI. It can serve as a detour for bypassing the scar. Injured descending axons have been shown to sprout and rewire to propriospinal neurons, whose axons are located in the spared tissue and project into the lower denervated spinal cord [69, 74]. Also, the propriospinal interneurons can sprout to innervate new targets below the lesion. In addition, these neurons might regenerate better than the projection neurons, because of the shorter distance of the axon stump to the cell body. They have been shown to upregulate growth-associated proteins and have a high intrinsic capacity for plasticity [75]. In partial injury models, such as dorsal or lateral transection or contusion,

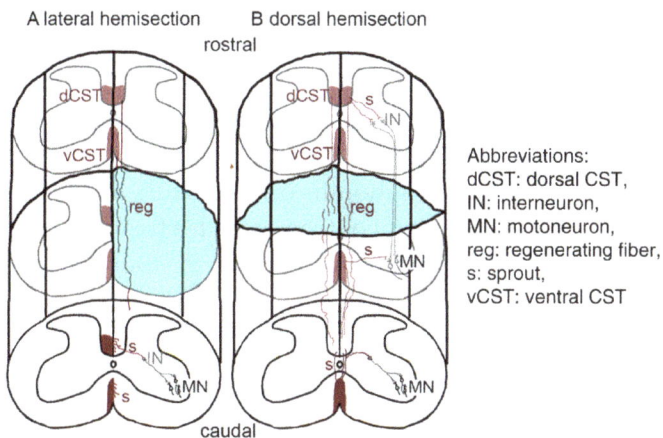

Figure 4 Axonal mechanisms leading to motor recovery exemplified for the dCST in two lesion models: (A) in the case of lateral Hx lesions, the contralateral intact dCST axons caudal to the lesion can sprout (s) and synapse with propriospinal interneurons (IN) connected to motoneurons (not necessarily at the same rostrocaudal level). The vCST on the intact side can also sprout to the ipsilateral side. Regeneration of the CST through the lesion is depicted by irregular lines since regenerating axons generally display a meandering and less straight course than the original tracts. (B) In the dorsal Hx model axons of the dCST can regenerate either through the lesion (irregular lines) or to form sprouts to make local connections with propriospinal interneurons whose axons run ventrally below the lesion and are connected to caudal motoneurons. The intact vCST can sprout and extend to the degenerated dCST tract or form new connections with interneurons that contact local motoneurons. Abbreviations: dCST: dorsal CST, IN: interneuron, MN: motoneuron, reg: regenerating fiber, s: sprout, vCST: ventral CST.

both regeneration from injured tracts and sprouting from spared tracts can be studied. It may be of importance to note that sprouting can be undirected, so that aberrant neuronal circuits may be formed [76]. Treatments can enhance sprouting and direct the sprouts to establish functional circuits.

5.2. Neuroprotection

After the primary insult, secondary damage due to, among others, inflammation, oxidative stress, and blood-brain barrier dysfunction causes the death of neurons (and glia) in the tissue surrounding the lesion [77]. The loss of local motor neurons leads to more extensive motor deficits in addition to the impairments caused by the injury to the descending motor tracts. The loss of spinal interneurons may disrupt intraspinal connections between motor centers. Therefore, a neuroprotective action of a treatment might, first, reduce functional impairments and, second, increase the possibility of local plasticity via interneurons (see Section 5.1.). For the analysis of neuroprotection, quantification of (moto-) neurons is performed at various distances rostrally and caudally from the lesion center [78]. A treatment could also lead to the protection of the brain and brainstem projection neurons from death or atrophy [8, 31, 79]. Quantification of the lesion size and spared white matter in standardized lesion models might also provide information about the protective effects of a treatment strategy.

6. Tracing and/or immunohistochemical (IHC) staining of motor and sensory tracts

The next step in SCI research is the histological analysis of regenerated axons. Short-term studies (up to several weeks after the injury) give information about early injury events, whereas long-term studies (up to several months or even years after the injury) are useful to investigate long-term effects and behavioral outcomes with a treatment compared to a control. In order to visualize regenerating axons from the specific spinal cord tracts, these can be marked via axonal tracing (Figure 3B) or detected by immunohistochemistry (IHC). In this section, the main techniques used in experimental SCI in rodents are summarized.

6.1. Tracing methods

6.1.1. Conventional tracing

Axonal tracing is an important tool for the investigation of regeneration after SCI (Figure 3B), holding the advantage that specific axonal populations are precisely marked. Conventional tracers label axons and neurons via the axonal transport [80]. Neuronal tracers can label the axons anterogradely (toward the axon terminal) which is the preferred method for analyzing their sprouting and regeneration. Retrogradely transported tracers (towards the cell body) are injected at the distal side of a lesion, in order to quantify the number of neurons with regenerated (distal) fibers and to visualize propriospinal neurons (see Section 6.4.).

Preferred application methods are pressure injection (liquid tracers), iontophoretic injection of electrically charged tracer molecules, or the insertion of dye crystals (carbocyanine dyes) [80]. The tracer can be detected via confocal microscopy using either its own fluorescence or IHC. The ideal survival time after the tracing depends on the tracer used, the distance between the site of tracer application and the area of interest, and the rate of its transport in the axons. A drawback of conventional tracing techniques is that in most cases not all axons of a neuronal population take up and transport the tracer substance. Many classical retrograde tracers are only, or more efficiently, taken up by injured axons and axon terminals, whereas the rate of the uptake by uninjured axons of passage is rather small. This can lead to nonspecific results [81].

Some examples for widely used monosynaptic neuronal tracers are the enzyme horseradish peroxidase, biotinylated dextran amine (BDA), and Fluoro Gold™. Examples of nonviral polysynaptic tracers are bacterial toxins, such as cholera toxin B. The drawback of nonviral polysynaptic tracers is, however, the dilution of signal after each synaptic step [82]. For the purpose of multisynaptic tracing, viral tracings are more suitable.

6.1.2. Viral tracings

When transneuronal tracing is desired, viral tracings are the method of choice. Transneuronal tracing is useful for the investigation of multisynaptic pathways and circuits [82]. The virus, which expresses a reporter gene in order to achieve the tracing, can replicate in the neurons and then infect other neurons which are connected via synapses. The virus replication further amplifies the signal, thereby avoiding the problem of signal dilution [8]. Very importantly, viral vector systems are very effective tools for gene therapeutic approaches. Frequently used viral systems used for axon tracing are adeno-associated viral vectors [83], lentiviral vectors [84], rabies virus [82], and herpes simplex virus [85]. The combination of viral tracings and gene therapy further offers the possibility to deliver a vector into specific areas.

A very elegant approach to investigate axonal pathways and their regeneration is the combination of viral tracing with optical tissue clearing and light sheet laser scanning microscopy [86–88].

6.2. Anterograde tracing of defined tracts

6.2.1. Motor cortex — CST tracing

In SCI research, the CST is the most established model tract for the investigation of regeneration and the associated locomotor functional outcome. Its origin in the sensorimotor cortex and its course through the pyramidal decussations and, in rodents, the dorsal center part of the spinal cord allow a very precise labeling and localization of the tract. By using a stereotactic frame, precise injections of the tracer of choice are applied into the sensorimotor cortex [8, 89]. In general, tracing is performed 2 (mice) to 3 (rats) weeks before sacrifice of the animals for histological analysis. In the case of BDA, tissue sections need to be stained with streptavidin coupled to a fluorescent marker. Fluorescently labeled BDA is available, but the signal is usually still enhanced by post-staining. Analysis is performed by confocal microscopy, counting regenerating axon profiles in and beyond the lesion site.

6.2.2. Nucleus ruber — RST tracing

The nucleus ruber can be traced in the same way as the CST; however, it is much smaller in size and therefore easier to miss [73].

6.2.3. Ascending sensory tracts: CTB tracing or CGRP staining

Cholera toxin β (CTB) is a tracer that is transported anterogradely, retrogradely and, as a recent study suggested, even transneuronally [90]. This tracer is used frequently to label the ascending sensory tracts in the dorsal column of the spinal cord. For this purpose, CTB is injected into the sciatic nerve that is crushed to achieve maximum uptake of the tracer [90]. This allows the specific analysis of the regeneration of ascending axons corresponding to the hindlimbs. In contrast, IHC staining for the marker calcitonin gene-related peptide CGRP allows the detection of axon profiles entering the spinal cord at all spinal segments. This, however, compromises the analysis of CGRP axons beyond the lesion, since axons from intact spinal levels above the lesion will also stain positively.

6.3. Raphespinal and coeruleospinal tracts

Because of their neurotransmitters serotonin (5-HT) and noradrenaline (NA), whose key synthesizing enzyme is tyrosine hydroxylase (TH), the tracts descending from the Raphe nuclei and locus coeruleus can be investigated by IHC using 5-HT- and TH-specific antibodies [73]. Since their fibers run both ventrally and dorsally, care should be taken to analyze only areas that are relevant to the localization of the lesion, for example, only the dorsal funiculus in case of a dorsal hemisection, with respect to regeneration. The possibility of sprouting from ventral axons cannot be ruled out, and some types of interneurons also express 5-HT.

6.4. Retrograde tracing

A very valuable tool for tracing regenerating neurons is retrograde tracing. When a tracer injected distally from the lesion site marks neurons proximally from the lesion site, these neurons have regenerated their fibers (provided the tracer is precisely located to the lesioned and not the spared region, and tracer diffusion can be ruled out). It can also answer the question whether axons from the intact side sprouted to the lesioned side. This technique was applied to show which brainstem nuclei were projecting into the distal cord [14] and to trace propriospinal interneuron networks [70]. If a retrograde tracer is applied to the spinal cord proximal to the lesion site, it can also be used to quantify the neurons "associated" with the lesion, for studying cell death or atrophy of neuronal populations [8].

7. Assessment of motor function

In order to assess motor recovery after experimental SCI and putative regenerative treatments, several functional tests are available. The choice of the tests depends not only on the lesion model but also on the costs, because some tests require specific commercial systems.

7.1. Basso, Beattie, and Bresnahan (BBB) locomotor score and subscore (rat) and Basso Mouse Scale (BMS, mouse)

The BBB open-field test, developed by Basso, Beattie, and Bresnahan [91], is an established test for the evaluation of hindlimb locomotor function of SCI rats. It is suitable for thoracic SCI models where it has become the first choice test to evaluate locomotor function [92]. The BBB score is based on the classification of hindlimb locomotor function using a scale which ranges from 0 (no spontaneous movement of the hindlimbs) to 21 (normal movement, coordinated walking pattern). For the evaluation procedure, the rats are placed in a defined open field where they are observed and evaluated by two trained observers. The animal's movements in the open field are scored over 4 minutes according to the criteria of the BBB locomotor rating scale [91]. The evaluation of coordination, an important parameter of the intermediate and late phases of the BBB, is not always clear without any doubt. This entails ratings in the medium-range scale intervals often leading to an artificial plateau. Therefore, and because usually not all aspects of locomotion are influenced by a treatment, the determination of a BBB subscore can be helpful to improve the sensitivity of the test [93]. Furthermore, additional automatic gait analysis helps to avoid potential subjective evaluation of coordination [94]. An advantage of the BBB locomotor rating scale is that preoperative training—which is a general requirement for many locomotor behavioral tests—is not necessary. However, as is generally the case for behavioral tests, preoperative handling of the experimental animals and their familiarization with the test surroundings are useful. Additionally, adaptations of the original BBB locomotor scale have been described also for severe thoracic injuries such as complete spinal cord transection [56, 95]. Since such severe lesions result in maximum BBB scores of 8–10, the spreading of the low and intermediate BBB values (BBB 1–10) allows a distinct evaluation of less prominent locomotor behavioral improvements.

The small size and rapid speed of mice caused investigators to develop a mouse-specific scale, the BMS [96]. The procedure of the animal walking in an open field is basically the same as described above, but parameters like coordination, paw position, and trunk instability are evaluated in a slightly different way than for rats. Similarly, for unilateral cervical SCI new locomotor rating scales have been developed, such as the forelimb locomotor assessment scale (FLAS) [97] or the forelimb locomotor scale (FLS) [98].

7.2. Horizontal ladder rung test and Gridwalk

The horizontal ladder walking test is used for the evaluation of fine motor control, coordination, and foot placing accuracy, all of which require certain degrees of sensory feedback. Therefore, this test is particularly useful for the investigation of locomotion after a thoracic CST injury. Video analyses of the runs allow the assessment of multiple parameters [99]. The mistakes the animals make during walking are evaluated and classified into predefined categories. The test apparatus consists of metal rungs (3 mm in diameter) placed between Plexiglas walls in predefined intervals (1–5 cm for rats). The spacing patterns should be regularly alternated to make sure that the animals' locomotor function and not their cognitive functions are evaluated. Care should be taken to provide gaps between the rungs that are neither too narrow (mistakes being made by an animal might not be observable) nor too large (the animal cannot walk across without fear of falling, or without having to jump between rungs). During pretraining, the animals learn to cross the horizontal ladder without interruption. Post-injury runs are recorded with a (high-speed) video camera from an angle slightly below the rod plane. This ensures the possibility to detect precise movements of all four paws and their digits. For evaluation, the predefined foot placing mistakes are counted. For mice, the procedure is similar, with smaller spacing (approximately 15 mm). For both species, several parameters of skilled walking can be observed, including correct placement, slight and deep slip, total miss, (partial) replacement, and correction [22, 99]. Alternative to the ladder test, the Gridwalk test makes use of grids to asses skilled walking.

7.3. Automated gait analysis methods

7.3.1. CatWalk™

The CatWalk™ system for automated quantitative gait analysis in SCI rats was developed by Hamers et al (2001). Classically, gait analysis in the form of footprint analyses has been (and still is by some groups) performed by painting the animal's paws with ink and letting it run on paper (or, an elegant variation, with developer and photographic paper) [100]. Static measures such as the distance between paws and toes could be measured, but no spatiotemporal resolution was achieved. The Catwalk™ system consists of a glass plate through which fluorescent light is internally reflected. When a mouse or rat places its paw on the glass, the light is deflected from the glass and the paw print lights up. The intensity is related to the pressure or weight support, which provides additional information about the functionality of the paw. A high-speed camera placed below the glass plate records all the runs (originally, a mirror projected the light toward the camera, but the commercial version (Noldus) images directly). A narrow walkway corridor on top of the glass plate ensures that the animals walk in a straight line. After a few days of habituation training, the animals walk steadily through the corridor. Recording is performed in the dark, but the commercial setup has a lid with red light above the walkway, so that the outline of the animal is visualized. After analysis, main parameters of interest are the stride length (step size), the base of support (distance between left and right paws), the walking speed, the duration of the swing and stand phase, the regularity index as a measure of coordination, and the intensity of the prints. Many more parameters can be studied, the choice of which can be based on the animal model [101, 102]. The CatWalk™ system has been used in the following SCI models: thoracic CST Tx, RST Tx, and dorsal Hx [8, 103]; thoracic contusion [101, 102]; pyramidotomy models [22]; and lateral cervical spinal cord contusion [104, 105], and in recent studies assessing the effects of training and gene therapy [106, 107]. The CatWalk™ can furthermore be combined with the horizontal ladder test by placing the ladder above the glass plate, so that footslips light up because the animal touches the glass plate [108].

7.3.2. Automated gait analysis using treadmill

The CatWalk™ is semi-automated, because the animals must voluntarily walk across the walkway and need pretraining. Again, scientists are striving to improve the existing systems (Neckel, 2015). New fully automated gait analysis platforms have been developed, including the DigiGait™ (Mouse Specifics, Inc.) [109–111] and the TreadScan™ (Clever Sys Incorporated) systems [112]. These two systems use transparent treadmills allowing the animals' gait analysis at constant speed, including the possibility to measure at different speeds.

7.3.3. MotoRater and kinematic analysis

The growing number of SCI models is accompanied by the need to modify the test systems. Recently, a new method for profiling locomotor recovery was developed in the lab of Martin Schwab [113]. This setup, now commercially available as the so-called MotoRater (TSE Systems), makes use of mirrors to image the mouse or rat that is walking in a Plexiglas basin from three sides (left, right, and below). The animals are tattooed on anatomical landmarks such as ilias crest, trochanter major of the hip, condylus lateralis of the knee, malleolus lateralis of the ankle, and the tip of the fifth toe. This way the walking is precisely monitored as stick diagrams and followed in time. As with the CatWalk™, the kinetics of even-ground walking patterns are analyzed. In contrast to the Catwalk, the researchers included new levels of difficulty in this system. A horizontal ladder is introduced to monitor precise paw placement and forelimb-hindlimb coordination. Alternatively, the basin is filled with water, either at levels where animals are wading (3 cm for rats, 1 cm for mice) or at levels where the animals have to swim. Wading brings the advantage that the water provides weight support. Furthermore, the animal's strength can be measured, because of the desire of the animal to raise its body as much as possible out of the water. In the original article, three types of SCI were compared (dorsal Hx, ventral Hx, and lateral Hx). For each lesion model, various aspects of the test revealed to be suitable in different ways. For example, skilled walking and overground locomotion are most suitable for the evaluation of thoracic dorsal Hx. For thoracic ventral Hx, wading was described to be the better test and for cervical lateral Hx, the authors observed improvement of hindlimb movements during wading and swimming. Due to the forepaw impairment, cervical Hx animals can hardly perform the ladder test and are poor at normal even-ground locomotion. Further studies of the same group made use of the MotoRater to assess the contribution of the brain stem nuclei to locomotor recovery [14] and the effects of training on motor skills after SCI [71].

Another kinematic gait analysis system makes use of reflective markers at essentially the same hallmarks as the MotoRater system (iliac crest, hip, knee, ankle, metatarsophalangeal joint, and toe). A motion capture system (SIMI Reality Motion Systems) is used to analyze gait parameters combined with electromyogram recording (EMG) [69, 70].

7.4. Sensory testing

Although less relevant than motor recovery, the recovery of sensory functions has a potential impact on locomotion. Furthermore, lesioned animals can develop neuropathic pain [114] which may be attenuated or, worse, aggravated by a treatment. Sensory tests performed after SCI include mechanical and nociceptive tests.

Sensorimotor reflexes can be tested by light touch to the paw, causing contact placing of the paw. Proprioceptive placing is elicited by stretching a tendon or joint [21]. Von Frey filaments are used to assess the animal's sensitivity to sub-threshold mechanical stimuli. For this purpose, filaments of increasing thickness are applied to the foot sole, exerting a defined force. This is normally not painful to the animal, so that only animals that suffer from mechanical allodynia (pain reaction from a normally non-painful stimulus) withdraw their paw from the filament. The minimum force eliciting a pain response is scored as paw withdrawal threshold [115]. Electronic versions of this test are available commercially (e.g., IITC Life Science, Ugo Basile). For the assessment of cutaneous hyperalgesia (increased pain from a pain-provoking stimulus), a hot plate or a commercial Plantar Test setup (e.g., Hargreaves Apparatus, Ugo Basil) [116] is used. The paw of interest is placed on a source of radiant heat or, in the case of the Planar Test, an infrared beam is precisely aimed at the central part of the animal's sole. The paw withdrawal time is recorded. Each paw is tested three times since the animal can also withdraw the paw spontaneously. Compared to the traditional hot plate test setup, the Plantar Test has the advantage of an automated, and therefore, accurate end-point detection [116].

For the majority of the sensory tests, the animal has to be able to move (withdraw) the paw. They can, therefore, generally not be performed with severely and completely spinal cord-injured animals that often lack the ability to perform limb movements below the level of the injury. For severely injured animals, the tail-flick test, a modification of the plantar hot plate test where the base of the tail is heated, can be applied [92].

7.5. Forelimb tests

For cervical hemisection lesions and for pyramidotomy, specific tests to analyze forelimb motor recovery have been developed [21]. Since these lesions are usually one-sided, the healthy side serves as an internal control. First, new locomotor rating scales (alternatives for the BBB) have been developed, such as the forelimb locomotor assessment scale (FLAS) [97] or the forelimb locomotor scale (FLS) [98]. Second, broad tests for paw preference are applied, such as the cylinder test, where the choice of the weight-bearing forelimb is monitored [22], and the grooming test, where the preferred paw for grooming is scored. Popular tests assessing dexterity include pasta eating or the Irvine, Beatti, Bresneham (IBB) forelimb rating scale, where the forelimb function is assessed, while the rat is eating a round-shaped cereal [117]. Furthermore, tests for the assessment of fine finger movements include the single pellet-grasping test or the staircase test [21, 71]. In these skilled forepaw tests, mice or rats have to reach for and grasp sugar pellets through a slit in a Plexiglas wall or from wells in a staircase setup (Lafayette Instruments (rat), Campden Instruments (mouse)). Video analyses of the sessions allow the assessment of multiple parameters. Some groups use the horizontal ladder as well to score forepaw locomotion, but the animals are usually poor at performing this test.

To further quantify grip a commercial grip strength meter is available (TSE Systems, Ugo Basile, Columbus Instruments), or the ability of the animal to keep its balance and hold on stably to an inclined plane (or cage grid) is measured.

7.6. Important considerations for functional testing

Several studies indicate that the choice of the motor tests should be based on the type of injury and the degree of impairment [113, 118]. For thoracic dorsal Hx, the horizontal ladder test and CatWalk™ gait analysis systems are suitable since even-ground walking and skilled walking are impaired, but display recovery over time. In the case of ventral Hx, the wading and swimming paradigms in the MotoRater provide more useful information on impairment and recovery. Cervical lateral Hx animals also perform better during wading and swimming. With regard to swimming, an assessment tool was developed in Sweden, where parameters like fore- and hindlimb usage, hindlimb alternation and position, trunk instability, body angle, and tail movements are precisely scored [119].

Care should, however, always be taken with the evaluation of the results. Animals can develop compensation strategies to perform a task in a different way than before the injury [118]. For example, animals primarily use their hindlimbs for swimming, but after a thoracic injury, they utilize their forelimbs. Therefore, distance or speed may recover, but the actual functional recovery of the hindlimbs might be still impaired. Another example is the grasping of food pellets that animals with forelimb impairment cannot do. Some animals tend to successfully develop a scooping strategy to retrieve pellets [118]. Investigators should be aware of this and monitor the strategies the animals use. The use of video equipment to accompany a test is therefore advisable.

The strain of the animals (and even the substrain produced by different suppliers) also plays an important role. Some animal strains perform better than others in tests which require the acquisition of certain skills [118, 120]. For example, in the staircase-skilled forepaw reaching test, Lister-hooded and Long-Evans rats perform much better than Lewis rats and Fischer rats [121, 122]. Housing is also of importance, since the amount of motor activity in the cage can provide training effects. This might mask a treatment effect, because the spontaneous recovery due to training may be too prominent. A popular cage enrichment in the form of sunflower seeds might compromise skilled grasping tests [118]. On the contrary, if the chosen test is too difficult for the animals in view of their impairment, recovery of function might be missed too. Other variables like circadian rhythms and stress can introduce variability. Therefore, it is vital to habituate the animals to the experimenters, to perform pre-injury recordings of the basal performance of the animals in the tests and to perform testing always at the same time of day under the same circumstances.

8. Discussion and conclusions

This chapter provides an overview of the main rodent models, experimental treatment strategies, histological analysis methods, and motor tests that are available for the investigation of neuronal regeneration and locomotor function after experimental SCI. The choice of the appropriate model depends on the research question and on the type of human injury which the investigation is based on. There is ongoing controversy regarding the comparability of experimental blunt versus sharp lesions to the clinical situation of human patients. Contusion/ compression injuries are very suitable for studying human traumatic SCI. These types of injury maintain tissue continuity even in the most severe cases, which is also observed in the vast majority of human spinal cord traumata. However, spared tissue bridges might compromise the analysis of treatment effects in experimental SCI. Moreover, blunt force spinal cord traumata are often accompanied by sharp lesions like maceration, laceration, or transection, for example by bone splinters. Therefore, sharp transections are also valid models, not least because they are easier to control and reproduce.

SCI experiments in rodents are essential for the development of new treatment strategies. They aim to extensively test treatment effects on multiple nerve tracts, to elucidate their mechanisms of action and, using multiple motor and sensory tests, to shed light on their ability to restore function. It is highly important to know whether a treatment is effective via neuroprotection, spared axon sprouting, or axon regeneration, since this will influence the choice of treatment that suits the patient best. Patients with incomplete lesions may benefit from plasticity-inducing treatments, whereas patients suffering from complete injuries require therapeutic strategies that induce regeneration. Patients with contusion lesions or complete injuries might further benefit from matrix or stem cell implantation to fill up cavities. When a treatment strategy displays promising effects in rodent SCI models, the next step will be to test it in a model system that is more close to human patients. In primates, the CST projects mainly dorsolaterally and originates from both left and right motor cortex, because a number of CST axons decussate along the spinal cord midline. These axons are capable of forming detour circuits reconnecting the motor cortex with denervated spinal cord areas in monkeys with lateral cervical Hx [123–125]. Due to the comparability with the anatomy of humans, the nonhuman primate cervical Hx model has been proposed to be a suitable model to test the recovery of forelimb skills after SCI [126].

Rodent research provided numerous important insights into the SCI field. To name a few, the regeneration and/or sprouting responses of tracts involved in locomotion, the involvement of the propriospinal system, the CPG circuits, and the ability to stimulate these without supra-spinal input all contributed to a better understanding of human spinal cord pathophysiology. Numerous treatments have been tested and have provided even more insights into how the various systems can be manipulated. However, to date, despite many years of extensive research, there are no clinical standard therapies for SCI which significantly increase the regenerative response to such a degree that they achieve strong (locomotor) improvements in human patients. This reflects the complexity of SCI. Although many treatments did not reach the clinic, they have been of enormous value to understanding the mechanisms of regeneration leading to functional motor recovery.

Author details

Christina F. Vogelaar[1*] and Veronica Estrada[2]

*Address all correspondence to: tineke.vogelaar@unimedizin-mainz.de

1 Institute of Microanatomy and Neurobiology, Johannes Gutenberg-University, Mainz, Germany

2 Molecular Neurobiology Laboratory, Department of Neurology, Heinrich-Heine-University, Duesseldorf, Germany

References

[1] Abbott A. Biomedicine: the changing face of primate research. Nature. 2014;506(7486): 24–6.

[2] Watson C, Harvey AR. Projections from the brain to the spinal cord 168. In: Watson C, Paxinos G, Kayalioglu G, editors. The Spinal Cord. A Christopher and Dana Reeve Foundation Text and Atlas. 1st ed. London: Academic Press; 2009. pp. 168–74.

[3] Du Beau A, Shakya Shrestha S, Bannatyne BA, Jalicy SM, Linnen S, Maxwell DJ. Neurotransmitter phenotypes of descending systems in the rat lumbar spinal cord. Neuroscience. 2012;227:67–79.

[4] Kayalioglu G. Projections from the spinal cord to the brain. In: Watson C, Paxinos G, Kayalioglu G, editors. The Spinal Cord. A Christopher and Dana Reeve Foundation Text and Atlas. 1st ed. London: Academic Press; 2009. pp. 148–58.

[5] Conta AC, Stelzner DJ. The propriospinal system. In: Watson C, Paxinos G, Kayalioglu G, editors. The Spinal Cord. A Christopher and Dana Reeve Foundation Text and Atlas. 1st ed. London: Academic Press; 2009. pp. 180–6.

[6] Slawinska U, Miazga K, Jordan LM. The role of serotonin in the control of locomotor movements and strategies for restoring locomotion after spinal cord injury. Acta Neurobiologiae Experimentalis. 2014;74(2):172–87.

[7] Ghosh M, Pearse DD. The role of the serotonergic system in locomotor recovery after spinal cord injury. Front Neural Circuits. 2014;8:151.

[8] Klapka N, Hermanns S, Straten G, Masanneck C, Duis S, Hamers FP, et al. Suppression of fibrous scarring in spinal cord injury of rat promotes long-distance regeneration of corticospinal tract axons, rescue of primary motoneurons in somatosensory cortex and significant functional recovery. The European Journal of Neuroscience. 2005;22(12): 3047–58.

[9] Vogelaar CF, Konig B, Krafft S, Estrada V, Brazda N, Ziegler B, et al. Pharmacological suppression of CNS scarring by deferoxamine reduces lesion volume and increases regeneration in an in vitro model for astroglial-fibrotic scarring and in rat spinal cord injury in vivo. PLoS One. 2015;10(7):e0134371.

[10] Hill RL, Zhang YP, Burke DA, Devries WH, Zhang Y, Magnuson DS, et al. Anatomical and functional outcomes following a precise, graded, dorsal laceration spinal cord injury in C57BL/6 mice. Journal of Neurotrauma. 2009;26(1):1–15.

[11] Zhang YP, Walker MJ, Shields LB, Wang X, Walker CL, Xu XM, et al. Controlled cervical laceration injury in mice. Journal of Visualized Experiments: JoVE. 2013;75:e50030.

[12] Hermanns S, Klapka N, Muller HW. The collagenous lesion scar—an obstacle for axonal regeneration in brain and spinal cord injury. Restorative Neurology and Neuroscience. 2001;19(1–2):139–48.

[13] Silver J, Miller JH. Regeneration beyond the glial scar. Nature Reviews Neuroscience. 2004;5(2):146–56.

[14] Zörner B, Bachmann LC, Filli L, Kapitza S, Gullo M, Bolliger M, et al. Chasing central nervous system plasticity: the brainstem's contribution to locomotor recovery in rats with spinal cord injury. Brain. 2014;137(Pt 6):1716–32.

[15] Mantilla CB, Greising SM, Stowe JM, Zhan WZ, Sieck GC. TrkB kinase activity is critical for recovery of respiratory function after cervical spinal cord hemisection. Experimental Neurology. 2014;261:190–5.

[16] Surey S, Berry M, Logan A, Bicknell R, Ahmed Z. Differential cavitation, angiogenesis and wound-healing responses in injured mouse and rat spinal cords. Neuroscience. 2014;275:62–80.

[17] Young W. Spinal cord contusion models. Progress in Brain Research. 2002;137:231–55.

[18] Jakeman LB, Guan Z, Wei P, Ponnappan R, Dzwonczyk R, Popovich PG, et al. Traumatic spinal cord injury produced by controlled contusion in mouse. Journal of Neurotrauma. 2000;17(4):299–319.

[19] Stokes BT, Jakeman LB. Experimental modelling of human spinal cord injury: a model that crosses the species barrier and mimics the spectrum of human cytopathology. Spinal Cord. 2002;40(3):101–9.

[20] Lee JH, Streijger F, Tigchelaar S, Maloon M, Liu J, Tetzlaff W, et al. A contusive model of unilateral cervical spinal cord injury using the infinite horizon impactor. Journal of Visualized Experiments: JoVE. 2012;65.

[21] Geissler SA, Schmidt CE, Schallert T. Rodent models and behavioral outcomes of cervical spinal cord injury. Journal of Spine. 2013;Suppl. 4. DOI: 10.4172/2165-7939.S4-001

[22] Starkey ML, Barritt AW, Yip PK, Davies M, Hamers FP, McMahon SB, et al. Assessing behavioural function following a pyramidotomy lesion of the corticospinal tract in adult mice. Experimental Neurology. 2005;195(2):524–39.

[23] Lang C, Bradley PM, Jacobi A, Kerschensteiner M, Bareyre FM. STAT3 promotes corticospinal remodelling and functional recovery after spinal cord injury. EMBO Reports. 2013;14(10):931–7.

[24] Moonen G, Satkunendrarajah K, Wilcox JT, Badner A, Mothe A, Foltz W, et al. A new acute impact-compression lumbar spinal cord injury model in the rodent. Journal of Neurotrauma. 2016;33(3):278–89.

[25] Wen J, Sun D, Tan J, Young W. A consistent, quantifiable, and graded rat lumbosacral spinal cord injury model. Journal of Neurotrauma. 2015;32(12):875–92.

[26] Inoue T, Lin A, Ma X, McKenna SL, Creasey GH, Manley GT, et al. Combined SCI and TBI: recovery of forelimb function after unilateral cervical spinal cord injury (SCI) is retarded by contralateral traumatic brain injury (TBI), and ipsilateral TBI balances the effects of SCI on paw placement. Experimental Neurology. 2013;248:136–47.

[27] del Mar N, von Buttlar X, Yu AS, Guley NH, Reiner A, Honig MG. A novel closed-body model of spinal cord injury caused by high-pressure air blasts produces extensive axonal injury and motor impairments. Experimental Neurology. 2015;271:53–71.

[28] Opatz J, Kury P, Schiwy N, Jarve A, Estrada V, Brazda N, et al. SDF-1 stimulates neurite growth on inhibitory CNS myelin. Molecular and Cellular Neuroscience. 2009;40(2): 293–300.

[29] Lu R, Schmidtko A. Direct intrathecal drug delivery in mice for detecting in vivo effects of cGMP on pain processing. In: Krieg T, Lukowski R, editors. Methods in Molecular Biology. Guanylate Cyclase and Cyclic GMP. Springer Link, Humana Press; 2013. pp. 215–21. DOI: 10.1007/978-1-62703-459-3_14

[30] DeVos SL, Miller TM. Direct intraventricular delivery of drugs to the rodent central nervous system. Journal of Visualized Experiments: JoVE. 2013;75:e50326.

[31] Carter LM, Starkey ML, Akrimi SF, Davies M, McMahon SB, Bradbury EJ. The yellow fluorescent protein (YFP-H) mouse reveals neuroprotection as a novel mechanism underlying chondroitinase ABC-mediated repair after spinal cord injury. The Journal of Neuroscience. 2008;28(52):14107–20.

[32] David S, Aguayo AJ. Axonal elongation into peripheral nervous system "bridges" after central nervous system injury in adult rats. Science. 1981;214(4523):931–3.

[33] Bunge MB. Bridging the transected or contused adult rat spinal cord with Schwann cell and olfactory ensheathing glia transplants. Progress in Brain Research. 2002;137:275–82.

[34] Tso D, McKinnon RD. Cell replacement therapy for central nervous system diseases. Neural Regeneration Research. 2015;10(9):1356–8.

[35] Papastefanaki F, Matsas R. From demyelination to remyelination: the road toward therapies for spinal cord injury. Glia. 2015;63(7):1101–25.

[36] Jin Y, Bouyer J, Shumsky JS, Haas C, Fischer I. Transplantation of neural progenitor cells in chronic spinal cord injury. Neuroscience. 2016;320:69–82.

[37] Slawinska U, Miazga K, Jordan LM. The role of serotonin in the control of locomotor movements and strategies for restoring locomotion after spinal cord injury. Acta Neurobiologiae Experimentalis. 2014;74(2):172–87.

[38] Sharp KG, Yee KM, Steward O. A re-assessment of long distance growth and connectivity of neural stem cells after severe spinal cord injury. Experimental Neurology. 2014;257:186–204.

[39] Lu P, Wang Y, Graham L, McHale K, Gao M, Wu D, et al. Long-distance growth and connectivity of neural stem cells after severe spinal cord injury. Cell. 2012;150(6):1264–73.

[40] Lu Y, Wang MY. Neural stem cell grafts for complete spinal cord injury. Neurosurgery. 2012;71(6):N13–5.

[41] Chen CT, Foo NH, Liu WS, Chen SH. Infusion of human umbilical cord blood cells ameliorates hind limb dysfunction in experimental spinal cord injury through anti-inflammatory, vasculogenic and neurotrophic mechanisms. Pediatrics and Neonatology. 2008;49(3):77–83.

[42] Schira J, Gasis M, Estrada V, Hendricks M, Schmitz C, Trapp T, et al. Significant clinical, neuropathological and behavioural recovery from acute spinal cord trauma by transplantation of a well-defined somatic stem cell from human umbilical cord blood. Brain. 2012;135(Pt 2):431–46.

[43] Schira J, Falkenberg H, Hendricks M, Waldera-Lupa DM, Kogler G, Meyer HE, et al. Characterization of regenerative phenotype of unrestricted somatic stem cells (USSC) from human umbilical cord blood (hUCB) by functional secretome analysis. Molecular and Cellular Proteomics. 2015;14(10):2630–43.

[44] Jones LL, Oudega M, Bunge MB, Tuszynski MH. Neurotrophic factors, cellular bridges and gene therapy for spinal cord injury. The Journal of Physiology. 2001;533(Pt 1):83–9.

[45] Samadikuchaksaraei A. An overview of tissue engineering approaches for management of spinal cord injuries. Journal of NeuroEngineering and Rehabilitation. 2007;4:15.

[46] Markakis EA, Redmond DE, Jr. Know thyself: autologous cell transplantation strategies for brain repair. Experimental Neurology. 2005;196(1):6–8.

[47] Ori S, Okada Y, Nishimura S, Sasaki T, Itakura G, Kobayashi Y, et al. Long-term safety issues of iPSC-based cell therapy in a spinal cord injury model: oncogenic transformation with epithelial-mesenchymal transition. Stem Cell Reports. 2015;4(3):360–73.

[48] Estrada V, Tekinay A, Muller HW. Neural ECM mimetics. Progress in Brain Research. 2014;214:391–413.

[49] Bakshi A, Fisher O, Dagci T, Himes BT, Fischer I, Lowman A. Mechanically engineered hydrogel scaffolds for axonal growth and angiogenesis after transplantation in spinal cord injury. Journal of Neurosurgery: Spine. 2004;1(3):322–9.

[50] Cai J, Ziemba KS, Smith GM, Jin Y. Evaluation of cellular organization and axonal regeneration through linear PLA foam implants in acute and chronic spinal cord injury. Journal of Biomedical Materials Research Part A. 2007;83(2):512–20.

[51] Novikova LN, Novikov LN, Kellerth JO. Biopolymers and biodegradable smart implants for tissue regeneration after spinal cord injury. Current Opinion in Neurology. 2003;16(6):711–5.

[52] Friedman JA, Windebank AJ, Moore MJ, Spinner RJ, Currier BL, Yaszemski MJ. Biodegradable polymer grafts for surgical repair of the injured spinal cord. Neurosurgery. 2002;51(3):742–51.

[53] Horn EM, Beaumont M, Shu XZ, Harvey A, Prestwich GD, Horn KM, et al. Influence of cross-linked hyaluronic acid hydrogels on neurite outgrowth and recovery from spinal cord injury. Journal of Neurosurgery: Spine. 2007;6(2):133–40.

[54] Prang P, Muller R, Eljaouhari A, Heckmann K, Kunz W, Weber T, et al. The promotion of oriented axonal regrowth in the injured spinal cord by alginate-based anisotropic capillary hydrogels. Biomaterials. 2006;27(19):3560–9.

[55] Tysseling-Mattiace VM, Sahni V, Niece KL, Birch D, Czeisler C, Fehlings MG, et al. Self-assembling nanofibers inhibit glial scar formation and promote axon elongation after spinal cord injury. The Journal of Neuroscience. 2008;28(14):3814–23.

[56] Estrada V, Brazda N, Schmitz C, Heller S, Blazyca H, Martini R, et al. Long-lasting significant functional improvement in chronic severe spinal cord injury following scar resection and polyethylene glycol implantation. Neurobiology of Disease. 2014;67:165–79.

[57] Brazda N, Voss C, Estrada V, Lodin H, Weinrich N, Seide K, et al. A mechanical microconnector system for restoration of tissue continuity and long-term drug application into the injured spinal cord. Biomaterials. 2013;34(38):10056–64.

[58] Haan N, Song B. Therapeutic application of electric fields in the injured nervous system. Advances in Skin and Wound Care (New Rochelle). 2014;3(2):156–65.

[59]   Singh B, Xu QG, Franz CK, Zhang R, Dalton C, Gordon T, et al. Accelerated axon outgrowth, guidance, and target reinnervation across nerve transection gaps following a brief electrical stimulation paradigm. Journal of Neurosurgery. 2012;116(3):498–512.

[60]   Young W. Electrical stimulation and motor recovery. Cell Transplant. 2015;24(3):429–46.

[61]   van den Brand R, Heutschi J, Barraud Q, DiGiovanna J, Bartholdi K, Huerlimann M, et al. Restoring voluntary control of locomotion after paralyzing spinal cord injury. Science. 2012;336(6085):1182–5.

[62]   Lavrov I, Gerasimenko Y, Burdick J, Zhong H, Roy RR, Edgerton VR. Integrating multiple sensory systems to modulate neural networks controlling posture. Journal of Neurophysiology. 2015;114(6):3306–14.

[63]   Wenger N, Moraud EM, Gandar J, Musienko P, Capogrosso M, Baud L, et al. Spatio-temporal neuromodulation therapies engaging muscle synergies improve motor control after spinal cord injury. Nature Medicine. 2016;22(2):138–45.

[64]   McPherson JG, Miller RR, Perlmutter SI. Targeted, activity-dependent spinal stimulation produces long-lasting motor recovery in chronic cervical spinal cord injury. Proceedings of the National Academy of Sciences U S A. 2015;112(39):12193–8.

[65]   Angeli CA, Edgerton VR, Gerasimenko YP, Harkema SJ. Altering spinal cord excitability enables voluntary movements after chronic complete paralysis in humans. Brain. 2014;137(Pt 5):1394–409.

[66]   Koopmans GC, Brans M, Gomez-Pinilla F, Duis S, Gispen WH, Torres-Aleman I, et al. Circulating insulin-like growth factor I and functional recovery from spinal cord injury under enriched housing conditions. The European Journal of Neuroscience. 2006;23(4):1035–46.

[67]   Lankhorst AJ, ter Laak MP, van Laar TJ, van Meeteren NL, de Groot JC, Schrama LH, et al. Effects of enriched housing on functional recovery after spinal cord contusive injury in the adult rat. Journal of Neurotrauma. 2001;18(2):203–15.

[68]   Fouad K, Tetzlaff W. Rehabilitative training and plasticity following spinal cord injury. Experimental Neurology. 2012;235(1):91–9.

[69]   Courtine G, Song B, Roy RR, Zhong H, Herrmann JE, Ao Y, et al. Recovery of supra-spinal control of stepping via indirect propriospinal relay connections after spinal cord injury. Nature Medicine. 2008;14(1):69–74.

[70]   Shah PK, Garcia-Alias G, Choe J, Gad P, Gerasimenko Y, Tillakaratne N, et al. Use of quadrupedal step training to re-engage spinal interneuronal networks and improve locomotor function after spinal cord injury. Brain. 2013;136(Pt 11):3362–77.

[71]   Starkey ML, Bleul C, Kasper H, Mosberger AC, Zorner B, Giger S, et al. High-impact, self-motivated training within an enriched environment with single animal tracking

dose-dependently promotes motor skill acquisition and functional recovery. Neurore-habilitation and Neural Repair. 2014;28(6):594–605.

[72] Sharp KG, Duarte JE, Gebrekristos B, Perez S, Steward O, Reinkensmeyer DJ. Robotic rehabilitator of the rodent upper extremity: a system and method for assessing and training forelimb force production after neurological injury. Journal of Neurotrauma. 2016;33. DOI: 10.1089/neu.2015.3987

[73] Schiwy N, Brazda N, Muller HW. Enhanced regenerative axon growth of multiple fibre populations in traumatic spinal cord injury following scar-suppressing treatment. The European Journal of Neuroscience. 2009;30(8):1544–53.

[74] Filli L, Schwab ME. Structural and functional reorganization of propriospinal connec-tions promotes functional recovery after spinal cord injury. Neural Regeneration Research. 2015;10(4):509–13.

[75] Siebert JR, Middelton FA, Stelzner DJ. Intrinsic response of thoracic propriospinal neurons to axotomy. BMC Neuroscience. 2010;11:69.

[76] Beauparlant J, van den Brand R, Barraud Q, Friedli L, Musienko P, Dietz V, et al. Undirected compensatory plasticity contributes to neuronal dysfunction after severe spinal cord injury. Brain. 2013;136(Pt 11):3347–61.

[77] Onose G, Anghelescu A, Muresanu DF, Padure L, Haras MA, Chendreanu CO, et al. A review of published reports on neuroprotection in spinal cord injury. Spinal Cord. 2009;47(10):716–26.

[78] Samano C, Kaur J, Nistri A. A study of methylprednisolone neuroprotection against acute injury to the rat spinal cord in vitro. Neuroscience. 2016;315:136–49.

[79] Carter LM, McMahon SB, Bradbury EJ. Delayed treatment with chondroitinase ABC reverses chronic atrophy of rubrospinal neurons following spinal cord injury. Experi-mental Neurology. 2011;228(1):149–56.

[80] Oztas E. Neuronal tracing. Neuroanatomy. 2003;2:2–5.

[81] Huh Y, Oh MS, Leblanc P, Kim KS. Gene transfer in the nervous system and implica-tions for transsynaptic neuronal tracing. Expert Opinion on Biological Therapy. 2010;10(5):763–72.

[82] Ginger M, Haberl M, Conzelmann KK, Schwarz MK, Frick A. Revealing the secrets of neuronal circuits with recombinant rabies virus technology. Frontiers in Neural Circuits. 2013;7:2.

[83] Blits B, Derks S, Twisk J, Ehlert E, Prins J, Verhaagen J. Adeno-associated viral vector (AAV)-mediated gene transfer in the red nucleus of the adult rat brain: comparative analysis of the transduction properties of seven AAV serotypes and lentiviral vectors. The Journal of Neuroscience Methods. 2010;185(2):257–63.

[84] Parr-Brownlie LC, Bosch-Bouju C, Schoderboeck L, Sizemore RJ, Abraham WC, Hughes SM. Lentiviral vectors as tools to understand central nervous system biology in mammalian model organisms. Frontiers in Molecular Neuroscience. 2015;8:14.

[85] McGovern AE, Davis-Poynter N, Rakoczy J, Phipps S, Simmons DG, Mazzone SB. Anterograde neuronal circuit tracing using a genetically modified herpes simplex virus expressing EGFP. The Journal of Neuroscience Methods. 2012;209(1):158–67.

[86] Soderblom C, Lee DH, Dawood A, Carballosa M, Jimena Santamaria A, Benavides FD, et al. 3D imaging of axons in transparent spinal cords from rodents and nonhuman primates. eNeuro. 2015;2(2).

[87] Schwarz MK, Scherbarth A, Sprengel R, Engelhardt J, Theer P, Giese G. Fluorescent-protein stabilization and high-resolution imaging of cleared, intact mouse brains. PLoS One. 2015;10(5):e0124650.

[88] Ertürk A, Becker K, Jahrling N, Mauch CP, Hojer CD, Egen JG, et al. Three-dimensional imaging of solvent-cleared organs using 3DISCO. Nature Protocols. 2012;7(11):1983–95.

[89] Steward O, Zheng B, Ho C, Anderson K, Tessier-Lavigne M. The dorsolateral corticospinal tract in mice: an alternative route for corticospinal input to caudal segments following dorsal column lesions. The Journal of Comparative Neurology. 2004;472(4): 463–77.

[90] Lai BQ, Qiu XC, Zhang K, Zhang RY, Jin H, Li G, et al. Cholera toxin B subunit shows transneuronal tracing after injection in an injured sciatic nerve. PLoS One. 2015;10(12):e0144030.

[91] Basso DM, Beattie MS, Bresnahan JC. A sensitive and reliable locomotor rating scale for open field testing in rats. Journal of Neurotrauma. 1995;12(1):1–21.

[92] Sedy J, Urdzikova L, Jendelova P, Sykova E. Methods for behavioral testing of spinal cord injured rats. Neuroscience and Biobehavioral Reviews. 2008;32(3):550–80.

[93] Lankhorst AJ, Duis SE, ter Laak MP, Joosten EA, Hamers FP, Gispen WH. Functional recovery after central infusion of alpha-melanocyte-stimulating hormone in rats with spinal cord contusion injury. Journal of Neurotrauma. 1999;16(4):323–31.

[94] Koopmans GC, Deumens R, Honig WM, Hamers FP, Steinbusch HW, Joosten EA. The assessment of locomotor function in spinal cord injured rats: the importance of objective analysis of coordination. Journal of Neurotrauma. 2005;22(2):214–25.

[95] Antri M, Orsal D, Barthe JY. Locomotor recovery in the chronic spinal rat: effects of long-term treatment with a 5-HT2 agonist. The European Journal of Neuroscience. 2002;16(3):467–76.

[96] Basso DM, Fisher LC, Anderson AJ, Jakeman LB, McTigue DM, Popovich PG. Basso Mouse Scale for locomotion detects differences in recovery after spinal cord injury in five common mouse strains. Journal of Neurotrauma. 2006;23(5):635–59.

[97] Anderson KD, Sharp KG, Hofstadter M, Irvine KA, Murray M, Steward O. Forelimb locomotor assessment scale (FLAS): novel assessment of forelimb dysfunction after cervical spinal cord injury. Experimental Neurology. 2009;220(1):23–33.

[98] Singh A, Krisa L, Frederick KL, Sandrow-Feinberg H, Balasubramanian S, Stackhouse SK, et al. Forelimb locomotor rating scale for behavioral assessment of recovery after unilateral cervical spinal cord injury in rats. The Journal of Neuroscience Methods. 2014;226:124–31.

[99] Metz GA, Whishaw IQ. Cortical and subcortical lesions impair skilled walking in the ladder rung walking test: a new task to evaluate fore- and hindlimb stepping, placing, and co-ordination. The Journal of Neuroscience Methods. 2002;115(2):169–79.

[100] Vogelaar CF, Vrinten DH, Hoekman MF, Brakkee JH, Burbach JP, Hamers FP. Sciatic nerve regeneration in mice and rats: recovery of sensory innervation is followed by a slowly retreating neuropathic pain-like syndrome. Brain Research. 2004;1027(1–2):67–72.

[101] Hamers FP, Lankhorst AJ, van Laar TJ, Veldhuis WB, Gispen WH. Automated quantitative gait analysis during overground locomotion in the rat: its application to spinal cord contusion and transection injuries. Journal of Neurotrauma. 2001;18(2):187–201.

[102] Hamers FP, Koopmans GC, Joosten EA. CatWalk-assisted gait analysis in the assessment of spinal cord injury. Journal of Neurotrauma. 2006;23(3–4):537–48.

[103] Hendriks WT, Eggers R, Ruitenberg MJ, Blits B, Hamers FP, Verhaagen J, et al. Profound differences in spontaneous long-term functional recovery after defined spinal tract lesions in the rat. Journal of Neurotrauma. 2006;23(1):18–35.

[104] Gensel JC, Tovar CA, Hamers FP, Deibert RJ, Beattie MS, Bresnahan JC. Behavioral and histological characterization of unilateral cervical spinal cord contusion injury in rats. Journal of Neurotrauma. 2006;23(1):36–54.

[105] Cao Y, Shumsky JS, Sabol MA, Kushner RA, Strittmatter S, Hamers FP, et al. Nogo-66 receptor antagonist peptide (NEP1-40) administration promotes functional recovery and axonal growth after lateral funiculus injury in the adult rat. Neurorehabilitation and Neural Repair. 2008;22(3):262–78.

[106] Hou J, Nelson R, Nissim N, Parmer R, Thompson FJ, Bose P. Effect of combined treadmill training and magnetic stimulation on spasticity and gait impairments after cervical spinal cord injury. Journal of Neurotrauma. 2014;31(12):1088–106.

[107] Hayakawa K, Uchida S, Ogata T, Tanaka S, Kataoka K, Itaka K. Intrathecal injection of a therapeutic gene-containing polyplex to treat spinal cord injury. Journal of Controlled Release. 2015;197:1–9.

[108] Smith JM, Lunga P, Story D, Harris N, Le Belle J, James MF, et al. Inosine promotes recovery of skilled motor function in a model of focal brain injury. Brain. 2007;130(Pt 4):915–25.

[109] Neckel ND. Methods to quantify the velocity dependence of common gait measurements from automated rodent gait analysis devices. The Journal of Neuroscience Methods. 2015;253:244–53.

[110] Ek CJ, Habgood MD, Callaway JK, Dennis R, Dziegielewska KM, Johansson PA, et al. Spatio-temporal progression of grey and white matter damage following contusion injury in rat spinal cord. PLoS One. 2010;5(8):e12021.

[111] Zhang B, Bailey WM, Braun KJ, Gensel JC. Age decreases macrophage IL-10 expression: implications for functional recovery and tissue repair in spinal cord injury. Experimental Neurology. 2015;273:83–91.

[112] Beare JE, Morehouse JR, DeVries WH, Enzmann GU, Burke DA, Magnuson DS, et al. Gait analysis in normal and spinal contused mice using the TreadScan system. Journal of Neurotrauma. 2009;26(11):2045–56.

[113] Zörner B, Filli L, Starkey ML, Gonzenbach R, Kasper H, Rothlisberger M, et al. Profiling locomotor recovery: comprehensive quantification of impairments after CNS damage in rodents. Nature Methods. 2010;7(9):701–8.

[114] Gwak YS, Kang J, Unabia GC, Hulsebosch CE. Spatial and temporal activation of spinal glial cells: role of gliopathy in central neuropathic pain following spinal cord injury in rats. Experimental Neurology. 2012;234(2):362–72.

[115] Detloff MR, Fisher LC, Deibert RJ, Basso DM. Acute and chronic tactile sensory testing after spinal cord injury in rats. Journal of Visualized Experiments: JoVE. 2012;62:e3247.

[116] Hargreaves K, Dubner R, Brown F, Flores C, Joris J. A new and sensitive method for measuring thermal nociception in cutaneous hyperalgesia. Pain. 1988;32(1):77–88.

[117] Irvine KA, Ferguson AR, Mitchell KD, Beattie SB, Lin A, Stuck ED, et al. The Irvine, Beatties, and Bresnahan (IBB) Forelimb Recovery Scale: an assessment of reliability and validity. Frontiers in Neurology. 2014;5:116.

[118] Fouad K, Hurd C, Magnuson DS. Functional testing in animal models of spinal cord injury: not as straight forward as one would think. Frontiers in Integrative Neuroscience. 2013;7:85.

[119] Xu N, Akesson E, Holmberg L, Sundstrom E. A sensitive and reliable test instrument to assess swimming in rats with spinal cord injury. Behavioural Brain Research. 2015;291:172–83.

[120] Kjell J, Sandor K, Josephson A, Svensson CI, Abrams MB. Rat substrains differ in the magnitude of spontaneous locomotor recovery and in the development of mechanical

hypersensitivity after experimental spinal cord injury. Journal of Neurotrauma. 2013;30(21):1805–11.

[121] Nikkhah G, Rosenthal C, Hedrich HJ, Samii M. Differences in acquisition and full performance in skilled forelimb use as measured by the 'staircase test' in five rat strains. Behavioural Brain Research. 1998;92(1):85–95.

[122] Galtrey CM, Fawcett JW. Characterization of tests of functional recovery after median and ulnar nerve injury and repair in the rat forelimb. Journal of the Peripheral Nervous System. 2007;12(1):11–27.

[123] Rosenzweig ES, Courtine G, Jindrich DL, Brock JH, Ferguson AR, Strand SC, et al. Extensive spontaneous plasticity of corticospinal projections after primate spinal cord injury. Nature Neuroscience. 2010;13(12):1505–10.

[124] Nout YS, Ferguson AR, Strand SC, Moseanko R, Hawbecker S, Zdunowski S, et al. Methods for functional assessment after C7 spinal cord hemisection in the rhesus monkey. Neurorehabilitation and Neural Repair. 2012;26(6):556–69.

[125] Nout YS, Rosenzweig ES, Brock JH, Strand SC, Moseanko R, Hawbecker S, et al. Animal models of neurologic disorders: a nonhuman primate model of spinal cord injury. Neurotherapeutics. 2012;9(2):380–92.

[126] Friedli L, Rosenzweig ES, Barraud Q, Schubert M, Dominici N, Awai L, et al. Pronounced species divergence in corticospinal tract reorganization and functional recovery after lateralized spinal cord injury favors primates. Science Translational Medicine. 2015;7(302):302ra134.

[127] Kuypers HG, Ugolini G. Viruses as transneuronal tracers. Trends in Neurosciences. 1990;13(2):71–5.

Permissions

List of Contributors

Mokhtar Arazpour, Mohammad Ebrahim Mousavi and Maryam Maleki
Department of Orthotics and Prosthetics, University of Social Welfare and Rehabilitation Sciences, Tehran, Iran

Guive Sharifi
Department of Neurosurgery, Shahid Beheshti University of Medical Sciences, Tehran, Iran

John V. Priestley and Adina T. Michael-Titus
Centre for Neuroscience and Trauma, Blizard Institute, Barts and The London School of Medicine and Dentistry, Queen Mary University of London, London, UK

Vanessa M. Doulames, Laura M. Marquardt, Bhavaani Jayaram, Christine D. Plant and Giles W. Plant
Department of Neurosurgery, Stanford University School of Medicine, Stanford, CA, USA

Victor S. Tapia and Juan Larrain
Center for Aging and Regeneration, Millennium Nucleus in Regenerative Biology, Faculty of Biological Sciences, Pontifical Catholic University of Chile, Santiago, Chile

Lenka Kresakova, Katarina Vdoviakova and Milan Cizek
University of Veterinary Medicine and Pharmacy in Kosice, Slovakia

Dasa Cizkova and Adriana-Natalia Murgoci
University of Veterinary Medicine and Pharmacy in Kosice, Slovakia

Laboratoire Protéomique, Réponse Inflammatoire et Spectrométrie de Masse (PRISM), Université Lille 1, Lille, France
Institute of Neuroimmunology, Slovak Academy of Sciences, Bratislava, Slovakia

Jusal Quanico, Isabelle Fournier and Michel Salzet
Laboratoire Protéomique, Réponse Inflammatoire et Spectrométrie de Masse (PRISM), Université Lille 1, Lille, France

Tomas Smolek and Veronika Cubinkova
Institute of Neuroimmunology, Slovak Academy of Sciences, Bratislava, Slovakia

Lucia Slovinska, Juraj Blasko, Miriam Nagyova, Eva Szekiova and Dasa Cizkova
Institute of Neurobiology, Slovak Academy of Sciences, Kosice, Slovakia

Monireh Ahmadi Bani, Mohammad Ebrahim Mousavi, Mahmood Bahramizadeh and Mohammad Ali Mardani
Department of Orthotics and Prosthetics, University of Social Welfare and Rehabilitation Sciences, Tehran, Iran

Christina F. Vogelaar
Institute of Microanatomy and Neurobiology, Johannes Gutenberg-University, Mainz, Germany

Veronica Estrada
Molecular Neurobiology Laboratory, Department of Neurology, Heinrich-Heine-University, Duesseldorf, Germany

Index

www.ingramcontent.com/pod-product-compliance
Lightning Source LLC
Chambersburg PA
CBHW070151240326

41458CB00126B/2965